Clubfoot

CURRENT PROBLEMS IN ORTHOPAEDICS

This series of monographs, each written or edited by a distinguished
authority, deals with special topics in orthopaedics, particularly those which
present major problems in diagnosis and management, and where recent
research advances carry important implications for patient care.

Already published

Menelaus: The Orthopaedic Management of Spina Bifida Cystica,
(2nd Edition)
Sevitt: Bone Repair and Fracture Healing in Man

In preparation

Dandy: Arthroscopic Surgery of the Knee
Leffert: The Brachial Plexus
Catterall: Legg-Calvé-Perthes Disease
Galasko, Bauer & Weber: Radionuclide Scintography in
Orthopaedics
Ling: Complications of Total Hip Replacement
Samuelson & Freeman: Surgical Treatment of the Arthritic
Ankle and Foot

Clubfoot

Vincent J. Turco, M.D.

Chief of Orthopaedic Surgery,
St. Francis Hospital, Hartford, Connecticut.

Assistant Professor of Orthopaedics,
University of Connecticut School of Medicine, Farmington, Connecticut.

Chief of Foot Clinic,
Newington Children's Hospital, Newington, Connecticut.

CHURCHILL LIVINGSTONE
NEW YORK EDINBURGH LONDON AND MELBOURNE 1981

Distributed in the United Kingdom by Churchill
Livingstone, Robert Stevenson House, 1-3 Baxter's
Place, Leith Walk, Edinburgh EH1 3AF and by
associated companies, branches and representatives
throughout the world.

First published in 1981

Printed in USA

ISBN 0-443-08033-X

9 8 7 6 5 4 3 2 1

Library of Congress Cataloging in Publication Data

Turco, Vincent J.
  Clubfoot.

  Bibliography: p.
  Includes index.
1. Clubfoot.   I. Title.
RD783.T87   617'.585   81-10109
ISBN 0-443-08033-X   AACR2

Dedication

This book is dedicated to my wife Gloria, my constant supporter and stimulus, and to Vincent Jr., Claudia, Paul and Monica.

Preface

Since my first exposure to pediatric orthopaedic surgery I was intrigued by the clubfoot deformity. After starting in practice my interest was further stimulated by the realization that in many cases the then accepted methods of treatment failed to achieve lasting corrections. In spite of years of treatment with manipulations, casts, braces, innumerable office visits and multiple operative procedures, the results left much to be desired. As patients were followed beyond skeletal maturity I learned that the triple arthrodesis was not a satisfactory solution. This experience provided the stimulus gradually to revise my method of treating this notoriously difficult problem. The assessment of results reveals that many acceptable results still leave much to be desired; this should stimulate us to elevate our goals and strive to attain the ideal of a near normal foot.

A review of the voluminous literature shows there is still great divergence of opinion regarding the etiology, pathological anatomy and treatment. It would be impossible to include every concept and method of treatment. A brief summary of some of the accepted concepts and methods of treatment is presented; for details the reader is referred to the original articles by the respective authors. Reasons will be given why certain methods of treatment have been discarded.

The etiology, diagnosis, pathological anatomy, radiologic examination and treatment of the idiopathic clubfoot are presented in detail. The normal anatomy and mechanics are reviewed in depth in order to establish the rationale of treatment. The differential diagnosis and pitfalls of the treatment of nonidiopathic clubfoot are discussed. The data are based on a life-time experience with clubfoot including the first patients I treated who are now adults. I found great advantage in being able to correlate the results to the clinical, x-ray and operative findings in children that were followed from birth to maturity. The cooperation of parents of private patients provided an excellent opportunity to evaluate both good and unsatisfactory results.

With so many divergent views it is easy to be controversial on a subject such as congenital clubfoot; this is not intended. I am very much aware of and respect the contributions made by many investigators regarding the etiology, pathology and treatment of this condition.

The purpose of this monograph is to serve as a guide for the practicing orthopaedist who sees an occasional clubfoot but has not had the luxury of enough long-term follow-ups to profit from his experience and alter his treatment. Hopefully, by using the methods of treatment and management as a guide, the surgeon should be able to obtain a satisfactory result and avoid iatrogenic complications and unrewarding prolonged treatment modalities. In the management I intend to report in detail the diagnosis and treatment of the resistant clubfoot. In no way do I mean to imply that these are the only methods capable of obtaining satisfactory results. The present methods of management—including both the non-operative and surgical treatment—were evolved after years of trial and error and the fortunate opportunity to observe the results of various methods of treatment, including the long-term results of my own patients. The emphasis is on the management of the resistant clubfoot and will include a long-term statistical analysis of the results, complications, and unusual findings in a large personal series of operative procedures and patients followed from birth to maturity.

In reviewing the voluminous literature on clubfoot it was obvious that succeeding generations rediscovered contributions that had been made by predecessors only to be discarded. The material to be presented represents the contributions of innumerable investigators. In the words of Montaigne—"I have here only made a nosegay of culled flowers, and have brought nothing of my own but the thread that ties them together."

Acknowledgments

Having finished this work I now understand and appreciate fully why many authors dedicate their books to their families. This work would never have been completed, or would have fallen far short of its mark, without the continued sacrifice and understanding of my family.

I single out with gratitude and empathy the many clubfooted children and their persevering parents. My hope is that the knowledge gained from their suffering will lessen the problem for future generations.

I am most grateful to my associates, Dr. Albert Casale and Dr. Anthony Spinella, for reading the manuscript and for their advice and help in making it possible for me to devote the time to this book; to Carol Turco, Cindy Duncan and Betsey Hill, my faithful staff, whose interest, cooperation and hard work made caring for the children affected with foot deformities a pleasure; to Diane Kycia for typing the manuscript; to Brooke Dramer of Churchill Livingstone for editing the manuscript; to Robert Martin, Frank Sullo, Joseph Milhomans and Mark Saccente in the photography department of St. Francis Hospital and Medical Center, Hartford, Connecticut; to Ruth Carroll and staff of the medical library of St. Francis Hospital and Medical Center; to Ann Williams of the outpatient clinic, St. Francis Hospital and Medical Center; to Charlotte Bryant, Lois Nelson, William Halpin and Janet Hall in the foot clinic at Newington Children's Hospital, Newington, Connecticut, and to the photography department, Newington Children's Hospital.

To Doctors P. V. C. Dingman and Martin Karno go my special thanks for their helpful suggestions and invaluable assistance in the preparation of this work.

Vincent J. Turco, M.D.

Introduction

"Clubfoot," "Piede torto," "Pie Bot," "Pie Zambo," Pé Eqüinovaro Congenito, "Klumpfuss" are worldwide synonyms for talipes equinovarus—a congenital deformity that has continued to plague the medical profession since before the days of Hippocrates. While much progress has been made since the 3rd century BC, confusion and divergent opinions regarding the etiology, pathogenesis, treatment and prognosis still exist. Some of the reasons for the divergent opinions are the following: the indiscriminate use of the all-inclusive term "congenital clubfoot" to describe all equinovarus deformities, many conditions can produce a clubfoot deformity with similar structural changes, the abnormality develops during the period of rapid skeletal development, therefore it is especially difficult to distinguish secondary adapted changes from primary structural abnormality. A congenital clubfoot deformity may be the only abnormality, as seen in the idiopathic deformity, or the deformed foot may be a local manifestation of a systemic congenital syndrome such as arthrogryposis, meningomyelocele, muscular dystrophy. At birth the congenital foot deformities may appear similar to each other irrespective of the etiology. Most of the anatomical dissections of the congenital clubfoot deformities have been done on aborted fetuses and neonatal deaths of babies with meningomyelocele or multiple congenital anamolies. There have been very few postmortem examinations of the idiopathic clubfoot.

A clubfoot deformity may also be acquired after birth secondary to muscle imbalance as in cerebral palsy, muscular dystrophy, or poliomyelitis. An example of this is seen in the famous painting by the Spanish artist Ribera (1588-1656), "Pie Bot," which is hanging in the Louvre Museum; the subject is a boy with a right talipes equinovarus associated with a right-sided hemiplegia, obviously a victim of cerebral palsy.

Misconceptions regarding the etiology, pathology and efficacy of treatment have been perpetuated in the literature because of the failure to distinguish the idiopathic from the secondarily acquired deformities. An example of this is the popularity of Achilles tenotomy for "clubfoot" which was introduced to England by W. J. Little, who first described the relation of difficult labor, premature birth and cerebral palsy (Little's disease). Little himself had poliomyelitis as a child which resulted in a left talipes equinovarus deformity. In describing the technique of Achilles lengthening, Little wrote in 1839—"As I regard Stromeyer to be the regenerator of this important addition to our means of curing clubfoot, and having experienced in my own person the success of this method of treatment, corroborated by the numerous cases which I have cured by the same means, I shall here only briefly enumerate the principles recommended by Stromeyer to be followed." Since Little published his paper in 1839, all too often simple Achilles lengthening is still being recommended for the cure of all clubfeet.

The pathogenesis, response to treatment, and the prognosis of the idiopathic clubfoot are different from the clubfoot that is a local manifestation of a systemic neuromuscular condition or an acquired talipes equinovarus that develops after birth. The challenge is the early recognition of the cause of the deformity in order to initiate rational treatment and provide the family with a more accurate, realistic prognosis and in addition to avoid iatrogenic complications that result from errors of commission or omission during treatment of nonidiopathic clubfeet.

The solution to the problem is difficult because considerable variations exist even among the so-called idiopathic deformities. In this manuscript our main concern is with the pathomechanics and treatment of the congenital idiopathic variety of talipes equinovarus.

Contents

1. History   1

2. Etiology   5

3. Normal Anatomy of the Foot   17

4. Pathologic Anatomy   35

5. Radiology   59

6. Nonoperative Treatment   85

7. Operative Treatment   109

8. Nonidiopathic Clubfoot and Other Foot Deformities   167

Index   189

1 | History

The earliest documentation of clubfoot comes from the ancient Egyptians. Paintings on the walls of their ancient tombs depict the clubfoot deformity, and a statue of a diastrophic dwarf with a clubfoot can be found in the Tutankhamen collection. Archeologic investigators in Mexico revealed that the Aztecs recognized clubfoot, treating it with splints made from cactus leaves. Hippocrates first described the clubfoot deformity around 300 BC.

In the middle of the 17th century, Arcaeus, Pare, and Fabrig recommended repeated stretching by the use of mechanical corrective apparatuses, which gradually eliminated the deformity with a turn-buckle.

In the 18th century, Cheselden of England utilized repeated stretching and bandaging to maintain the correction. The bandage was made of "several pieces of linen rag dipt in a mixture of whites of egg and flour."

Scarpa[10] in 1803 described the pathologic anatomy in "A Memoir on the Congenital Clubfoot in Children." In this treatise he described the deformity as a "twisting of the scaphoid os calcis and cuboid around the astragalus," calling it a "congenital dislocation of the astragalo calcaneo scaphoid complex." Scarpa also described the contractures of the soft parts and devised an apparatus with springs in an attempt to stretch the contractures and reduce the scaphoid.

Subcutaneous tenotomy of the Achilles tendon was first performed by Lorenz in Frankfort in 1782. Delpech of France in 1823 reported the same technique in a few patients with acquired talipes equinovarus. In 1831, Stromeyer of Germany popularized subcutaneous tenotomy and performed the operation on Little,[8] who later introduced and popularized this method of Achilles tendon lengthening in England in 1839. Guérin in 1838 appears to have been the first to report the use of plaster of Paris in the treatment of clubfoot. In 1857, Solly performed one of the first bony operations for clubfoot—removal of part of the cuboid—which was a precursor of the present-day Dillwynn-Evans operation.

In 1866, Adams[1] differentiated the acquired talipes equinovarus from the congenital variety. He also noted that the head and neck of the talus were deviated

1

medially. He felt that this medial deviation of the talus was a secondary adaptive change and not a primary defect, and stated "the altered form is adaptive rather than result of the defective power of development."

Lund performed the first recorded talectomy for clubfoot in 1872. During the latter part of the 19th century, Hugh Thomas (of Thomas splint fame and an uncle of Sir Robert Jones) devised the Thomas wrench, which was used to forcibly manipulate and correct the deformity. After the manipulation, a splint was applied to hold the correction. This method was used either alone or following surgery; fortunately, this brutal method was discontinued.

Except for tenotomy of the Achilles tendon, the operative treatment of the clubfoot began in 1867 with Lister's introduction of aseptic technique and the discovery of anesthesia. These landmark discoveries, along with the introduction of the Esmarch Tourniquet in 1873, which permitted bloodless surgery, increased interest in the surgical approach. The introduction of the pneumatic tourniquet by Cushing, in 1904, reduced the danger of tourniquet palsies and made surgery of the extremity less hazardous and more popular.

In 1890 Phelps, an orthopedist in New York City, described a one-stage medial-plantar soft-tissue release with lengthening of the tendons. He also did an osteotomy of the neck of the talus with wedge resection of the calcaneus.

In 1898, Walshingham and Hughes renewed interest in the theory that the deformity was due to a germ plasm defect of the head of the talus. They, along with others, reported osteotomy of the talus as a means of correction. Years later Elmslie in 1920[6] and Denis Browne in 1937[4] once again recommended osteotomy of the neck of the talus to correct the deformity.

In 1906, Codvilla[5] from Italy described a soft-tissue release with lengthening of the tendons, including the anterior tibial. Codvilla made a plea for soft-tissue surgery to be done when a child is about three years of age. This plea was made at a time when the prevalent methods of treatment were excochleation bony operations of the calcaneus and cuboid.

From 1900 to 1930, many varied operations were recommended for the surgical correction of clubfoot. In addition, during this period considerable progress was made in our knowledge of the pathologic anatomy of this deformity.

In 1930, Hiram Kite[7] popularized nonoperative treatment with serial manipulations and plaster cast immobilization. Kite was a great advocate of nonoperative treatment and stressed the need for gentle manipulations.

In his classic monograph in 1930, Brockman[3] described the morbid anatomy of clubfoot as a "congenital atresia of the astragalo-calcaneo-scaphoid joint." He also described a two-stage soft-tissue release for correction.

In 1934 Denis Browne renewed interest in mechanical intrauterine pressure as a cause of the deformity. He advised forceful manipulations before the application of his Denis Browne splint. Forceful manipulations have since fallen into disrepute because most now feel this method causes deformity of the bones and stiffness of the joints.

McCauley,[9] in 1947, made significant contributions to our knowledge and treatment of the resistant foot. He noted: "all tend to recur except those completely corrected, readily in a few months." McCauley was one of the first to stress radiographic evaluation of the results of treatment. A half century after the discovery of the roentgen ray, McCauley stated: "X-ray standards of correction are more reliable than clinical appearance." In 1960, Bost[2] stressed the importance of releasing the contracted plantar structures.

Currently, all agree that nonoperative treatment is best and should be attempted before considering surgery. In recent years, there has been more emphasis on earlier surgical correction, and many varied surgical techniques have been recommended. The multiplicity of operations and methods of treatment are ample evidence that the correction of clubfoot is still an unsolved problem.

Notably absent in the literature are the reasons why certain methods of treatment have been discarded. In reviewing the history of clubfoot, one is impressed by the fact that succeeding generations rediscover the forgotten contributions of our predecessors and time and again present them as something new.

While much progress has been made since the days of Hippocrates, there are still many unsolved mysteries regarding clubfoot. Hopefully, by adding the contributions of many recent investigators to the knowledge made available to us by our predecessors and critically analyzing our results, especially the failures, future victims of congenital clubfoot will reap the benefits.

REFERENCES

1. Adams, W: Clubfoot: Its Causes Pathology and Treatment. J. & A. Churchill, London, 1866.
2. Bost, F. C., Schottstadt, E. R., and Larsen, L. J.: Plantar dissection—an operation to release the soft tissues in recurrent talipes equinovarus. Journal of Bone and Joint Surgery, *42A:*15, 1960.
3. Brockman, E. P.: Congenital Clubfoot. J. Wright and Sons, Bristol, 1930.
4. Browne, Denis: Talipes equinovarus. Lancet, *2:*969, 1934.
5. Codvilla, A.: Sulla cura del piede equino varo congenito: Nuovo metodo di cura cruenta. Archivo Orthopedica, *23:*245, 1906.
6. Elmslie, R. C.: Principles in treatment of congenital talipes equinovarus. Journal of Orthopedic Surgery, *2:*119, 1920.
7. Kite, J. H.: The Clubfoot. Grune & Stratton, New York, 1964.
8. Little, W. J.: A Treatise on the Nature of Clubfoot and Analogous Distortions. W. Jeffs, S. Highley, London, 1839.
9. McCauley, J. C., Jr.: Operative treatment of club feet. New York State Journal of Medicine, *47P:*255, 1947.
10. Scarpa, A.: Memoir on Congenital Clubfeet. (Translated from Italian.) A. Constable, Edinburgh, 1818.

2 | Etiology

While our knowledge of the pathologic anatomy and treatment of clubfoot have increased through the years, the etiology of the idiopathic congenital form of this deformity is still unknown and remains an unsolved mystery.

Through the years, many theories have been proposed, discarded, rediscovered, and represented with renewed enthusiasm by succeeding investigators. During the past 200 years, the same basic concepts of etiology, with slight modifications, have enjoyed temporary acceptance as the solution to the unsolved puzzle.

Among the many factors responsible for the number of dissenting opinions on etiology is the frequent confusion of the terms genetic and congenital. A *congenital* abnormality simply indicates that a child is born with a defect—the abnormality is produced by pathologic changes in the normal developmental process of the embryo. A congenital deformity may result from an inborn genetic defect at the time of conception, or from adverse factors in the uterine environment, affecting normal embryologic development. In a *genetic* condition, the potential is passed on to succeeding generations. Many genetic syndromes are not congenital but manifest themselves after birth, as for example, muscular dystrophy.

Confusion also exists because many different etiologic factors can produce similiar, but not necessarily identical, foot deformities. Teratologic and congenital defects differ from each other because the end result is determined not only by the nature of the intrauterine trauma but also, and more importantly, by the stage of embryologic development at the time the insult occurs. Thus, the same factor is capable of producing varying deformities, depending on when the insult occurs. For example, after the first trimester, the insult may have little effect on fetal development.

Some of the changes noticed at birth may be primary or acquired, in part, during intrauterine growth and development. At birth, it may be difficult to distinguish primary changes from abnormalities acquired secondarily, especially if the congenital anomaly occurs early in fetal development. Since growth and development of the musculoskeletal system continue after birth, this statement can be extended to include postnatal acquired changes, as seen in neurologic problems and muscular dystrophies. The inability to differentiate between acquired and primary changes, and the failure to realize that some abnormal findings are the effect and not the cause of the deformity, have contributed to the disagreement regarding etiology.

Further confusion exists because the term clubfoot has been used to describe all talipes equinovarus deformities, regardless of the cause. The diagnosis "congenital clubfoot" describes a deformity noted at birth and includes idiopathic and nonidiopathic talipes equinovarus. In the nonidiopathic clubfoot, the deformity is a local manifestation of a systemic skeletal syndrome; the foot deformity and the associated skeletal anomalies are due to the same etiologic factor that caused the failure of normal fetal development. The nonidiopathic clubfoot can result (1) from muscle imbalance, as in neuromuscular conditions; (2) from fibrosis of soft parts, as seen in arthrogryposis; or (3) from bone and joint anomalies. In the idiopathic clubfoot, the foot is the only deformity; the musculoskeletal system is otherwise normal.

THEORETICAL CONSIDERATIONS

Many theories have been advanced to explain the etiology of idiopathic clubfoot. When examined closely, however, the evidence supporting each theory falls short on some vital point. Through the years, the following theories have been suggested by many investigators: (1) mechanical factors in utero; (2) neuromuscular defect; (3) primary germ plasm defect; (4) arrested fetal development; (5) heredity; and (6) heredity and environment combined.

Mechanical Factors in Utero

The mechanical theory is the oldest theory and was first proposed by Hippocrates.[8] He believed that the foot was held in a position of equinovarus by external uterine compression. Some investigators have expressed the opinion that uterine pressure is increased by diminution of amniotic fluid, as in oligohydramnios. Proponents of this theory[3,20] maintain that the lack of uterine liquor prevents fetal movement and makes the fetus vulnerable to extrinsic pressures.

Most investigators have concluded that it is hardly likely that intrauterine pressure would consistently cause the same type of deformity limited to the foot. Those opposed to this mechanical theory also point out that, during the first months of pregnancy when the fetus is forming, it is floating in amniotic fluid. They maintain that the absence of an increased incidence of clubfoot in pregnancies with an overcrowded uterus (twinning, large babies, hydramnios, and primiparous uteri) would negate the theory that increased intrauterine compression is an important etiologic factor. However, one still cannot rule out the possibility that a transient elevation of intrauterine pressure at a vulnerable time could interfere with the normal development of the foot.

Neuromuscular Defect

Some investigators maintain that the equinovarus foot is always the result of neuromuscular defects. Recently, Issacs and coworkers[11] did histochemical and electron microscopic studies of the extrinsic muscles of 60 clubfeet in patients less than 5 years old. Their study "indicated a dominant neurogenic factor in the causation." They were of the opinion that muscle imbalance may produce the deformity, particularly if the imbalance develops at an early stage of intrauterine development. The authors also stated: "We believe that clubfoot is a resistant form of arthrogryposis multiplex congenita and clinically the legs of the patient with clubfeet may be indistinguishable from those of arthrogryposis." On the contrary, Ionasecu et al.[10] did biochemical and electron microscopy studies on gastrocnemius muscle biopsies from five patients with idiopathic clubfeet (aged 1½ to 10 years), and 20 normal controls. They concluded that: "Fibrosis in severe idiopathic clubfeet may be a major factor in maintaining deformity by limiting the amount of stretch the calf muscles can undergo during growth. However, the fibrosis should not be considered as a primary etiologic factor.[11] Others have reported studies of the histology of muscles and clubfeet and recorded no abnormality.[12,23,26] At birth, the appearance of the clubfoot deformity in arthrogryposis or muscular dystrophy may be indistinguishable from the idiopathic clubfoot. It is not known whether the changes in the muscle structure are the cause or the result of the deformity, or whether they are primarily or secondarily acquired.

There are many factors that make a neurogenic cause unlikely. The association of clubfoot with spina bifida is well known; however, it is unlikely that a neurologic disorder is primarily responsible for all idiopathic deformities because:

1. Not all children with spina bifida have clubfoot.
2. The deformities associated with congenital neurologic defects do not present with the same constant characteristics of the idiopathic clubfoot.
3. The neurologically deformed foot is usually more flexible than the rigid congenital idiopathic foot.
4. In neurologic problems, the clubfoot usually can be placed in dorsiflexion.
5. In neurologic problems, plantar-flexed talus and talipes calcaneovalgus are more common than talipes equinovarus.
6. In general, neuromuscular deformities due to cerebral palsy and muscular dystrophy can be stretched and shown to respond temporarily to manipulation, unlike the majority of clubfeet.

Weak peroneal muscles have also been incriminated. It has been suggested that peroneal nerve palsy may develop as a result of pressure exerted by the flexed fetal knee on the mother's pelvis.[25] However, electromyographic studies by Orofino[16] and Takasy[24] have shown no lower motor neuron lesions.

Ritsillä[21] produced talipes equinovarus deformities in rabbits by tenodesis, by tendon resection, and by ligament transection followed by immobilization in equinus. He concluded: "The results of the present study confirm the importance of considering primary soft tissue changes as a factor provoking secondary skeletal deformities." Again, however, the unanswered question is: What is the primary cause of soft-tissue contractures?

Primary Germ Plasm Defect

Irani and Sherman[12] have suggested that the deformity probably results from a primary germ plasm defect, affecting the head and neck of the talus. They dissected 11 extremities with talipes equinovarus and 14 normal feet. All were from stillbirths of 22 to 36 weeks gestation or neonatal deaths. In their anatomic dissection they found

> no primary abnormalities of the vessels, nerves, muscles and tendon insertions. The most conspicuous and the only constant abnormality is found in the anterior part of the talus. The neck of the talus is always short. The anterior portion of the talus is always rotated in the medial and plantar direction so that the articular surface no longer faces directly forward. . . . Since the anlagen for the talus are fully formed at six weeks and the tarsal joints well developed at seven weeks. The changes to the embryo must occur before the seven weeks of intrauterine life. It is difficult to imagine an exogenus trauma which at this stage of development would damage only the anterior part of the talus—and often in one foot. Furthermore the hereditary aspect of the clubfoot deformity is hard to reconcile with exogenus trauma.

That a completely normal-shaped head and neck of the talus fails to develop after correction supports this theory.

Antagonists of the primary germ plasm defect theory have described the same abnormality of the talus, but they attribute it to secondary adaptive changes. It is not clear how one explains a unilateral deformity resulting from a genetic defect; nor is it known why only the head of the talus is involved, leaving the body of the talus unscathed. Further, one might ask why the deformity is corrected by realigning the navicular and calcaneus on the talus, without changing the medial angulation of the head and neck of the talus?

Arrested Fetal Development

Intrauterine Environment. In 1863, Heuter and von Volkman[7] first proposed that arrest of fetal development early in embryonic life was a cause of congenital clubfoot. They maintained that the malformation develops because early in embryonic life the physiologic developmental phase of the foot remained stationary. Other investigators have also reported a physiologic position in embryologic development during which the foot is similiar to talipes equinovarus. With normal development, the equinus diminishes as the foot gradually pronates to assume the normal position seen at birth. Many investigators have shown that equinus, varus, and adduction normally occur in the early stages of fetal development, and their studies of the pathologic anatomy of clubfoot have revealed that it resembles the embryonic foot at about 2 months of age.

Böhm[2] in 1929 wrote the classic paper supporting the theory of arrested fetal development. He and other proponents of this theory maintain that some factor in the uterine environment, at a critical stage in embryonal development, interferes with the normal development of the fetus, causing it to arrest during the stage the foot is normally in the physiologic equinovarus position. If this position is maintained beyond the normal period of time, the child develops a clubfoot.

In 1889, Bessel-Hagen,[1] on the basis of his investigations of embryonic feet, opposed the theory that during embryonic life there is a normal stage when the foot assumes the physiologic form of a clubfoot. Mau[14] in 1927 expressed the opinion that clubfoot cannot be due to arrested fetal development because "the embryonic foot does not show the distortion of the bones about the tarsal joints which is found in a clubfoot." Currently, many investigators feel that the hypothesis of arrested fetal development is a plausible embryologic explanation.

Recently, A. Victoria Diaz[6] from Spain reported a study of 59 human embryonic feet, ranging in size from 4.8 to 65 mm. The conclusion was that changes in the position of the embryonic feet, as well as movements of the talus and calcaneus, are due to a "spurt" in growth of the distal ends of the tibia and fibula. In the first stage (fibula phase), the calcaneus was pushed and displaced into the embryonic position (equinovarus). In the second stage (tibial phase), the talus was pushed and the foot pronated into the usual fetal position. Diaz theorized that, if growth were arrested temporarily during the "tibial phase" without the tibial growth spurt, the foot would remain in its embryonic position and the child would be born with a clubfoot. This mechanism would be comparable to the varus deformity that occurs with overgrowth of the fibula following epiphyseal injury of the medial malleolus in childhood. This interesting theory may receive some additional circumstantial support from the observation that many clubfeet do have an underdeveloped and less prominent medial malleolus. (Dr. E. J. Rothchild has observed one child with congenital clubfoot associated with an *absent* medial malleolus.) But once again the devil's advocate would ask: Is this cause or result?

Environmental Influences. The harmful environmental influence of teratogenic agents on fetal environment and development are well exemplified by the effects of rubella and Thalidomide early in pregnancy. In laboratory animals, many investigators have shown that harmful environmental influences can produce congenital abnormalities. The type of abnormality depends on timing in relation to the stage of embryonic development. No one, however, has been able to implicate any intrauterine toxic agent in a congenital deformity limited to the foot.

For obvious reasons, there have been no studies to support the hypothesis that maternal illness early in pregnancy is the causative factor. It is all too easy for a mother with a deformed child to think back and recall a possible disturbance in early pregnancy. On the other hand, it is just as easy to forget an illness that occurred 7 to 8 months earlier. In questioning intelligent mothers, I have been impressed with the significant number who recalled an unusual illness or bleeding early in pregnancy which had not occurred during their previous (or subsequent) pregnancies with normal children.

In the days before birth control pills and legalized abortion, I served as an orthopedic consultant to a home for unwed mothers. In this capacity, I saw all of the children born with orthopedic problems, and was impressed with the high incidence of clubfoot in this group. A 10-year review of all babies born in this institution revealed an incidence of one clubfooted child per 193 live births—an incidence 5 times more common than that in a community hospital in the same area with a similar population. These statistics, plus the clinical impressions noted earlier, should nevertheless be considered only as circumstantial evidence. However, they do raise questions regarding possible uterine environmental factors early in the pregnancies of teenage mothers.

Heredity

It is well known that clubfoot tends to be familial in a significant number of cases. Studies by Palmer,[18] Wynne-Davies,[27] and others[4,13,22,23] have shown that there is an increased incidence of clubfoot among relatives of affected probands, greatly exceeding the number expected by chance alone. One must therefore conclude that heredity plays some role in the etiology of clubfoot; however, the manner in which it contributes is unclear. Investigators have proposed contradictory genetic mechanisms, and the theories advanced have encompassed a broad spectrum of modes of inheritance that includes: autosomal recessive, sex-linked recessive, autosomal dominant, and multifactorial modes.[4,18,22,28]

None of the recent studies on genetics of idiopathic clubfoot has answered the questions raised by Idelberger[9] in his excellent study of 174 pairs of twins, 40 identical and 134 dizygotic, with clubfoot. Idelberger reported that 13 of 40 (33 percent) identical monozygous twins were concordant, whereas only 4 of 134 (3 percent) of dizygous twins were concordant. It is difficult to explain why 67 percent of the identical twins, enjoying the same uterine environment, were not affected; yet there was a significant increase as compared to fraternal twins.

It is now believed by most investigators that congenital idiopathic clubfoot is inherited as a polygenic multifactorial trait;[19,28] that is, whereas genetic factors are clearly important in clubfoot, the mode of inheritance is not a simple one. It is of interest to note that congenital dislocation of the hip (CDH), scoliosis, cleft palate, and myelomeningocele are all considered to have multifactorial inheritance, and that each has a similar incidence of about 1 per 1,000 live births. Why, however, is the incidence of CDH greater in females, while the reverse is true of congenital clubfoot? Palmer[19] has suggested that females require a greater number of predisposing factors than males to produce a clubfoot deformity.

In multifactorial inheritance, since many factors jointly cause the disorder, one might be more apt to see what looks like the same disease or abnormality occurring in a wide range of clinical variations. The polygenetic theory would explain why clubfoot deformities vary in their degrees of severity, resistance, and variations in pathologic anatomy. The clubfoot appears to be explicable on the basis of a multifactorial threshold hypothesis.

Heredity and Environment Combined

Many investigators agree that the deformity probably results from a combination of multifactorial genetic predisposition and some obscure intrauterine environ-

APPALACHIAN REGIONAL
HOSPITALS, INC.

PATIENT CHARGE II

NAME

DATE

BY

LIST DRUGS, FLUIDS, OXYGEN, ETC.

AMOUNT

ARHI
FORM F-V-26 (10-63)

mental factor. Wynne-Davies[28] states that polygenic inheritance is more susceptible to the influence of environmental factors, thereby supporting the theory of hereditary predisposition and environment. Further support of this combination theory is provided by Idelberger's study,[9] in which he reported that both twins of an identical set were affected (concordant) in 33 percent of cases. The combined hypothesis maintains that some intrauterine factor, in conjunction with hereditary predisposition, causes a disturbance in development at a critical stage of the embryonic development of the foot, thereby causing an arrest of normal fetal development.

Based on clinical experience, this author believes that most idiopathic clubfeet are attributable to an abnormality in fetal environment, affecting fetal development at a crucial stage; hereditary predisposition is probably an added factor in many cases.

However, this combination theory leaves many questions unanswered: Why are monozygous twins discordant? Why is the deformity unilateral? Why is there a greater incidence of clubfoot in males? Why does the same deformity occur so consistently with different etiologic agents? Why is the deformity localized to the foot?

GENETIC COUNSELING

It is difficult to give accurate genetic counseling in polygenic hereditary conditions, such as idiopathic clubfoot. According to Palmer,[18,19] Wynne-Davies,[29] and Scott,[22] the probability that another child with clubfoot will be born into a family with an affected child is 20 to 30 times greater than the accepted incidence of 1 in 1,000. When one of the parents has talipes equinovarus, the estimated risk is about 3 to 4 percent. When both parents are affected, there is an estimated 15 percent risk that they will have another child with clubfoot.[22] The predictability of this risk is quite different from that of clubfoot associated with diastrophic dwarfism, an autosomal recessive condition. In this condition, the risk of clubfoot would be 1 in 4.

It is not unusual for a mother to develop guilt feelings because she believes her child's deformity occurred as a result of some event during pregnancy for which she feels responsible. With empathy, the physician should allay these feelings of guilt and give her intelligent, realistic, and rational explanations based on current knowledge of the subject. These explanations should reassure her that the deformity was beyond her control. Another responsibility the physician has is to reassure the worried and often depressed parents that, with good treatment and considerable family cooperation, the child will not be "crippled for life" but will be able to lead a reasonably normal life, as a child and as an adult.

INCIDENCE OF CLUBFOOT

Most investigators have reported an incidence in talipes equinovarus of 1 to 2 per 1,000 live births. Based on a study of 1 million births at 1,160 hospitals in the United States for the year 1977,[5] the National Birth Defects Monitoring Program reported an incidence for clubfoot, without central nervous system anomalies, of 2.29 cases per 1,000 births. Clubfoot was found to be the most common congenital anomaly in this study. The incidence was slightly greater—2.77 per 1,000—in the northeastern section of the United States. This study also showed a slight decline in the rate of clubfoot in all regions of the country during the preceding 5 years.

Demographic Statistics

Demographic and racial studies have produced some interesting statistics to support the polygenic hereditary theory of etiology. A comprehensive study in Hawaii, by Chung et al.[4] has produced some meaningful statistics regarding the incidence among Caucasians, Hawaiians, and Orientals. Chung et al. noted no difference among Orientals (Chinese, Japanese, Filipinos, and Koreans). The Hawaiian study reported an overall incidence of clubfoot of 1.33 per 1,000 births, slightly higher than that reported by Wynne-Davies[28] for England (1 per 1,000 births). The incidence among the Caucasian population of Hawaii was similar to that of the English study; however, there was a significant difference in the incidence among the three racial groups: 6.8 per 1,000 live births in the Hawaiians, 1.12 per 1,000 in the Caucasians, and 0.56 per 1,000 in the Orientals. A major contribution of this study is that the statistics show that the risk and incidence of clubfoot appear to increase with the proportion of Hawaiian or Caucasian "blood" in mixed marriages with Orientals. Napoli[15] studied 471 patients with congenital clubfoot in São Paulo, Brasil, a city with more than 2 million Oriental inhabitants. Like the Hawaiian study, Napoli's study showed that the incidence of clubfoot was less common among Orientals, compared with the Caucasian population.

An increased incidence of clubfoot has also been reported among the Maoris of New Zealand, who, like the Hawaiians, are also Polynesian.[28] Perez-Teuffer[17] reported a higher incidence of clubfoot in Mexico, where talipes equinovarus represents 60 percent of all congenital anomalies. Clubfoot seems to be more prevalent in the Middle East[30] and countries on the Mediterranean coast of North Africa.

Personal Series

It is very difficult to get accurate figures regarding significant data from hospital charts and even certain statistical reports because many authors lump all foot deformities under the category "clubfoot." In addition, they do not differentiate between the localized idiopathic deformity and a general musculoskeletal syndrome.

I have reviewed my experience with 468 patients who were treated or seen in consultation through the years. Patients with deformities secondary to arthrogryposis, neuromuscular syndromes, and so on, were excluded.

Sex Ratio

In our series of 468 patients, there were 334 (71.36 percent) males and 134 (28.63 percent) females, for a sex ratio of 2.5 males to 1 female (Table 2-1). Kite,[29] in his series of 1,509 cases, reported 70 percent males and 30 percent females.

TABLE 2-1. IDIOPATHIC CLUBFEET–SEX RATIO

Sex	Patients	
	Number	Percent
Male	334	71.36
Female	134	28.63
Total	468	99.99
Sex ratio	2.5 males to 1.0 females	

Laterality

All investigators have reported that over 50 percent of cases of clubfoot are bilateral deformities. In my series, 56.76 percent were bilateral; Chung reported bilaterality in 55.75 percent. In the unilateral group, Chung,[4] Kite,[13] and Palmer[18] all reported a slight preponderance of right side involvement. However, in his Hawaiian study, Chung could find no difference with respect to laterality among the three racial groups (Hawaiians, Caucasians, and Orientals). When we pooled their data, the right foot was involved in 53.76 percent. Our data on laterality revealed that the right and left sides were equally involved: right side, 104 patients; left side, 102 patients (Table 2-2). It is interesting that only 37 of the 262 bilateral deformities (14.12 percent) were corrected without surgery, suggesting the possibility that a bilateral deformity may be more resistant than a unilateral one.

Family History

It is very difficult to get accurate data on family history from public health statistics and hospital charts. A review of the literature reveals that the percentage of patients with a positive family history varies between a low of 5 percent and a high of 50 percent.[18] However, it must be pointed out that some of these studies included all types of congenital foot deformities. To the best of my knowledge, in my series of 468 patients there were 84 (17.9 percent) with a known positive family history. These data are accurate. What is unknown is how many more patients had relatives with a clubfoot deformity and were inaccurately reported to me as having a "negative family history."

In the group with a positive family history, 58 were male and 26 female, a ratio of 2.2 males to 1 female compared to the 2.5:1 incidence for the entire group. Fifty of the 84 deformities were bilateral, 60 percent compared to 56 percent for the entire group.

TABLE 2-2. LATERALITY

Side	No. of Patients	Percent
Bilateral	262	55.98
Right	104	22.22
Left	102	21.79
Total	468	99.99

TABLE 2-3. AFFECTED RELATIVES OF
PROBANDS WITH CLUBFEET*

Relationship	No. of Children†
Father	16
Mother	6
Sibling	20
Grandparent	4
Uncle	21
Aunt	10
First Cousin	26

* 19 children had more than one relative with a clubfoot
† 84 of 468 (17.9%) patients had a positive family history

In the 26 females with a positive family history, 14 (53 percent) had bilateral deformities; in the remaining 110 females with a negative family history, 33 (30 percent) had bilateral deformities. A higher incidence of bilaterality among females with a positive family history concurs with the statistics reported by Palmer,[18,19] Chung,[4] and Wynne-Davies.

Nineteen of the 84 patients with a positive family history had more than one relative with a clubfoot deformity. Twenty children had siblings with clubfeet; 22 were products of a clubfooted parent; and 4 had a parent and a sibling with clubfoot. (Table 2-3).

There were eight sets of twins: one monozygotic set and seven dizygotic sets. Both of the monozygotic twins were afflicted; one had a bilateral deformity while the cotwin had a unilateral deformity. Interestingly, among dizygotic twins, in no case were both twins affected with clubfoot. All of the dizygotic twins were mixed, except for one female whose cotwin sister was normal. In all mixed twins, the male was affected but his cotwin sister was normal.

SUMMARY

The etiology of idiopathic clubfoot is still unknown. However, from our present knowledge it would appear that no single theory of etiology can be implicated in all cases. This raises the possibility that all of the theoretical causes proposed can lead to an idiopathic clubfoot—a concept that would explain the many variations seen in congenital clubfoot insofar as appearance, resistance, response to treatment, and prognosis are concerned.

According to available data, the concensus is that heredity is an important factor in a significant percentage of cases. In a majority of cases, however, the family history is negative. It is plausible to theorize that in many cases a child inherits a polygenic predisposition which, together with intrauterine factors, leads to an arrest of the normal embryologic development of the foot. This theory agrees with the genetically acceptable one that polygenic conditions predispose to changes in the uterine environment.

In general, all agree that mechanical compression by the uterine wall per se is not a plausible explanation. However, intrauterine mechanical pressure, temporarily affecting early fetal development, could conceivably interfere with the normal growth and development of the foot.

In some cases, the neuromuscular hypotheses appear plausible. We have all seen cases that appear to be typical, idiopathic clubfeet at birth only to find out later that we are dealing with a deformity that is secondary to a muscular dystrophy or a neurologic problem that becomes evident postnatally. In large clinics, all too frequently one encounters the most recalcitrant clubfeet, which appear to be localized forms of arthrogryposis with the foot or feet being the only extremities involved.

In conclusion, no one theory can explain the etiology of all congenital idiopathic clubfeet. Evidence has been presented that different causative factors can produce the same deformity. Since one theory cannot be implicated as the sole cause in all cases, the possibility exists that idiopathic talipes equinovarus represents a deformity that can be caused by many etiologic agents, thereby explaining the variations encountered.

The answer regarding the etiology of clubfoot will depend on new advances in our knowledge of genetics and the development of more sophisticated histochemical and microscopic examinations of neuromuscular and collagen tissues.

REFERENCES

1. Bessell-Hagen, F.: Die Pathologie and Therapie des Klumpfusses. O. Petters, Heidelberg, 1889.
2. Böhm, M.: The embryologic origin of clubfoot. Journal of Bone and Joint Surgery, *9NOZ*:229, 1929.
3. Browne, D.: Congenital deformities of mechanical origin. Proceedings of the Royal Society of Medicine, *29:*1409, 1936.
4. Chung, C. S., Nemechek, R. W., Larsen, I. J., and Chung, G. H. S.: Genetic and epidemiological studies of clubfoot in Hawaii. Human Heredity, *19:*321, 1969.
5. Congenital Malformations Surveillance: Jan.–Dec. 1977. U.S. Dept. H.E.W., Public Health Service, Atlanta, Georgia.
6. Diaz, A. V.: Embryological contribution to the aetiopathology of Idiopathic clubfoot. Journal of Bone and Joint Surgery, *61B:*1979.
7. Heuter, and von Volkman. Zu der Frage üben das wesen des angeborenen klumpfüsses, Deutsch Klinik *15:*487, 1863.
8. Hippocrates. Francis Adams: The Genuine Works of Hippocrates. (Translated from Greek). Williams and Wilkins, Baltimore.
9. Idelberger, K.: Die Z. Willingspathologic des angeborenen klumpfusses. A. Orthop. *69:*1, 1939.
10. Ionasecu, V., Maynard, J. A., Ponsetti, V., and Zellweger, H.: Helvetica Paediatrica Acta, *29:*305, 1974.
11. Issacs, H., Handelsman, J. E., Badenhorst, M., and Pickering, A.: The muscles in

clubfoot—a histological histochemical and electron microscopic study. Journal of Bone and Joint Surgery, *59B:*000, 1977

12. Irani, R. N., and Sherman, M. S.: Pathological anatomy of clubfoot. Journal of Bone and Joint Surgery, *45A:*000, 1963.
13. Kite, J. H.: The Clubfoot. Grune and Stratton, New York, 1964.
14. Mau, C.: Der Klumpfuss. Ergebn, Chir. Orthop., *20:*000, 1927.
15. Napoli, M. M.: Tratamento Cirugico do pe' equinovaro congenito Recidivado e inveterado. Sao Paulo, Brasil, 1964.
16. Orofino, C. F.: The etiology of congenital clubfoot. Acta Orthopaedica Scandinavica *29:*000, 1959.
17. Perez-Teuffer, A.: 1975.
18. Palmer, R. M.: The genetics of talipes equinovarus. Journal of Bone and Joint Surgery, *46A:*542, 1964.
19. Palmer, R. M., Conneally, P. M., and Pao-LoYe, O. O.: Studies on the inheritance of idiopathic talipes equinovarus. Orthopedic Clinics of North America *5:*000, 1974.
20. Parker, R. W., and Shattoch, S. G.: The pathology and etiology of congenital clubfoot. Transactions of the Pathological Society of London, *35:*423, 1884.
21. Ritsilä, V. A.: Talipes equinovarus and vertical talus produced experimentally in newborn rabbits. Acta Orthopaedica Scandinavica, Suppl., *121:*000 1969.
22. Scott, C. I.: Genetic disorders in orthopaedic practice. American Academy of Orthopedic Surgeons, Institute Course Lecture, February, 1979.
23. Stewart, S. I.: Clubfoot; its incidence, cause and treatment. An anatomical-physiological study. Journal of Bone and Joint Surgery, *33A:*557, 1951.
24. Takasy, S.: Electromyographic study of congenital clubfoot. Journal of the Japanese Orthopedic Association *36:*857, 1900.
25. White, J. W.: The importance of the tibialis in the production and recurrence of clubfeet. Southern Medical Journal, *22:*675, 1929.
26. Wiley, A. M.: An anatomical and experimental study of muscle growth in clubfoot. Journal of Bone and Joint Surgery, *41B:*821, 1959.
27. Wynne-Davies, R.: Genetic and environmental factors in the etiology of TEV. Clinical Orthopaedics and Related Research, *84:*000, 1972.
28. Wynne-Davies, R.: Heritable Disorders in Orthopaedic Practice. Blackwell Scientific Publications, Oxford, 1973.
29. Wynne-Davies, R.: Family studies and the cause of congenital clubfoot. Journal of Bone and Joint Surgery, *46B:*000, 1964.
30. Youssef, A. S., Waly, H. T., Booz, M. K.: Treatment of talipes equinovarus. Journal of the Kuwait Medical Association, vol. 9, 1975.

3 | Normal Anatomy of the Foot

A thorough knowledge of the normal anatomy of the foot is essential to understanding clubfoot, a deformity that essentially represents a fixed exaggeration of the normal equinovarus position. Because the foot is such a complicated structure, involving multiple bones, articulations, muscles, and ligaments, any discussion of foot deformities must include the ankle joint. The foot and ankle should be considered together as one functional unit because of the interrelationship of the mechanics of the tibiotalar, subtalar, and midtarsal joints.

MUSCLES

The muscles of the lower leg and foot can be divided into two groups: *the extrinsic muscles,* which are a group of muscles that originate in the leg and insert on the bones of the foot, and *the intrinsic muscles,* which arise from the tarsal bones and insert on the bones of the foot or tendons of the extrinsic muscles.

The Extrinsic Muscles

The Gastrocnemius and the Soleus. Together, these form the muscle mass described as the triceps surae. The tendo Achillis, the common tendon of the triceps, inserts on the posterior tuberosity of the calcaneus. The triceps, which forms the greater part of the calf, is the powerful plantar flexor of the foot. When it contracts, it pulls the posterior tuberosity of the calcaneus upwards and, because the Achilles inserts on the calcaneus medial to the subtalar axis, it also inverts the foot.

The three remaining deep muscles of the calf, the flexor hallucis longus, the tibialis posterior, and the flexor digitorum longus, also contribute to the muscle mass of the calf.

The Flexor Hallucis Longus. This muscle, the more lateral of the three

17

deep muscles, arises from the lower two-thirds of the posterior surface of the fibula and the interosseous membrane. From its lateral origin, it runs obliquely downward and medially to form a tendon just above the ankle joint. The tendon of the flexor hallucis longus, which lies in a groove on the posterior surface of the tibia and the talus, continues under the sustentaculum tali of the calcaneus and then passes under the navicular, forward in the sole of the foot, to insert on the terminal phalanx of the big toe. Often, an additional slip runs to the flexor digitorum longus.

The Flexor Digitorum Longus.   The most medial of the three deep posterior muscles, the flexor digitorum longus, arises from the posterior surface of the tibia. Its tendon, which begins higher than that of the flexor hallucis longus, passes behind the medial malleolus below the posterior tibial tendon in a separate tunnel. It lies superficial to the deltoid ligament and runs into the sole of the foot under the navicular, where it crosses the hallucis longus. Distally, it is joined by the quadratus plantae (flexor accessorius), and divides into four tendons that insert on the terminal phalanges. The tendons of both long toe flexors are enclosed in separate, well-defined tendon sheaths.

The Master Knot of Henry.   This structure is a hypertrophied thickening of the tendon sheaths of the long toe flexors and functions as a suspensory ligament that holds the tendons of the flexor digitorum longus and the flexor hallucis longus close to the plantar surface of the navicular (like an annular ligament).[7] This fibrous tissue knot is located below the navicular tuberosity. It envelops the two tendons in separate tunnels at the point where the flexor hallucis longus crosses above the flexor digitorum longus. Distal to the knot, the tendons continue on to their respective insertions. They often send communicating slips to each other and for this reason, traction on either tendon often produces flexion of all the toes in unison.

The Tibialis Posterior.   A most important muscle in the clubfoot deformity, the tibialis posterior, lies between the flexor hallucis longus and the flexor digitorum longus. It arises from the lateral portion of posterior surface of the tibia, the undersurface of the interosseous membrane, and the adjacent fibula. The muscle belly extends downward and medially from its lateral origin, and in the lower fourth of the leg it becomes tendinous as it passes deep and then anterior to the flexor digitorum longus. Its tendon lies in a groove behind the medial malleolus, enclosed in a thickened sheath separate from the flexor digitorum longus. It then runs forward under the lacinate ligament superficial to the deltoid and passes distally along the medial plantar surface of the foot, where it has an extensive insertion on the tarsal and metatarsal bones. While the prime insertion of this tendon is on the tuberosity of the navicular, it also gives off fibrous expansions that insert on the sustentaculum tali of the calcaneus, the adjacent cuneiforms, the metatarsal, and the plantar calcanonavicular (spring) ligament.

The tibialis posterior muscle supinates (adduction and inversion) and plantar flexes the foot as it pulls the navicular medially and downward; the medial malleolus serves as its fulcrum. It is important to note that the only extrinsic muscles that insert on the calcaneus—i.e., the tibialis posterior and the triceps surae—both plantar flex and invert the heel. In applying knowledge of the normal anatomy of the foot to clubfoot surgery, it must be appreciated that the tibialis posterior insertion has a broad expansion that includes attachments to the sustentaculum tali of the calcaneus and the spring ligament in addition to its prime insertion on the navicular tuberosity. When the tibialis posterior is surgically transferred to the dorsum of the foot, it must be remembered that this muscle arises from the posterolateral aspect of the calf and runs medially in a course parallel to the tibialis anterior. In the distal third, the two muscles are separated by the interosseous membrane—hence the rationale for transferring the tibialis posterior muscle through the interosseous membrane, rather than medially around the medial malleolus of the tibia. Transplanting the posterior tibial anteriorly through the interosseous space permits the muscle transfer to pull in a straight line, rather than in a corkscrew course, around the medial malleolus, thereby fulfilling one of the prerequisites for a successful tendon transfer.

The Anterior Tibial. This muscle arises from the anterolateral surface of the tibia and the interosseous membrane and runs downward and medially under the extensor retinaculum to insert on the first cuneiform and on the base of the first metatarsal.

The Peroneus Longus and Peroneus Brevis. Both of these muscles arise from the lateral surface of the fibula. Their tendons pass behind the lateral malleolus; the brevis attaches to the base of the fifth metatarsal, whereas the peroneus longus tendon runs deep across the sole of the foot to attach to the base of the first metatarsal and the adjacent cuneiform. The peroneals pronate and plantar flex the foot.

The Intrinsic Muscles

These muscles are important in cases of clubfoot with a cavus deformity. For this discussion, the abductor hallucis, flexor digitorum brevis, abductor digiti quinti, and quadratus plantae (flexor accessorius) can be considered a common mass of muscle that arises in several successive layers from the medial and plantar surface of the tuberosity of the calcaneus and the plantar aponeurosis.

The Plantar Aponeurosis. This is essentially a strong superficial ligament that extends from the os calcis to the toes. The central part of the aponeurosis is much stronger and thicker than the medial portion, which covers the undersurface of the abductor hallucis.

The Abductor Hallucis. This is the longest muscle of this group. It lies along the medial border of the foot and covers the plantar nerves and vessels. The abductor hallucis arises from the most medial part of the calcaneus and runs along the medial border of the foot to form a tendon that inserts, together with the medial tendon of the flexor hallucis brevis, into the medial side of the proximal phalanx of the great toe.

BONES

The Tarsal Bones

The Calcaneus. The largest of the tarsal bones, the calcaneus [Fig. 3-1 *(A)*], articulates with the talus and the cuboid. On its superior surface, there are three

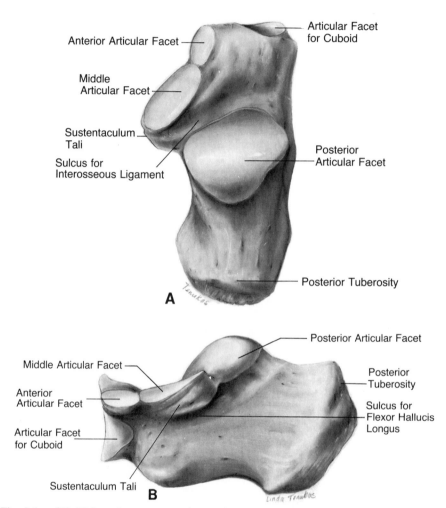

Anterior Articular Facet

Articular Facet for Cuboid

Middle Articular Facet

Sustentaculum Tali

Posterior Articular Facet

Sulcus for Interosseous Ligament

Posterior Tuberosity

A

Posterior Articular Facet

Middle Articular Facet

Posterior Tuberosity

Anterior Articular Facet

Sulcus for Flexor Hallucis Longus

Articular Facet for Cuboid

Sustentaculum Tali   **B**

Fig. 3-1.   *(A),* Right calcaneus, superior surface. The posterior convex facet supports the body of the talus and articulates with concave facet on the undersurface of the talus. The concave middle and anterior facets support proximal and lateral portions of the head of the talus. The calcaneal sulcus together with its counterpart on the undersurface of the talus form the tarsal canal, which contains the talocalcaneal interosseous ligament and divides the subtalar area into anterior and posterior compartments. *(B),* Right calcaneus, medial surface. The middle facet above the sustentaculum anterior to the sulcus supports the head and neck of the talus. The sustentaculum, an important landmark, provides bony attachment for the tibialis posterior, superficial deltoid, and the spring ligament, and also serves as a pulley to redirect the flexor hallucis in a lateral course. The length and downward inclination of the posterior tuberosity form a long lever arm to enhance the mechanical advantage for the Achilles attachment.

articular facets that support the talus: the posterior articular facet, which is convex, articulates with the concave facet under the body of the talus. Anterior to the posterior articular facet is the calcaneal sulcus, a groove on the superior surface of the calcaneus that lies below a similar sulcus (the talar sulcus) on the undersurface of the talus. Together these grooves form the tarsal canal, which contains the talocalcaneal interosseous ligament.

The tarsal canal expands laterally to form the sinus tarsi, a funnel-shaped canal whose medial narrow portion lies just above and posterior to the sustentaculum tali of the calcaneus. It runs laterally and forward to form the wide opening of the funnel just in front of the lateral malleolus (sinus tarsi). In front of the tarsal tunnel is the concave *middle articular facet,* which articulates with a corresponding facet on the undersurface of the head and neck of the talus. In front and slightly lateral to the middle articular facet is the *anterior articular facet,* which articulates with its counterpart on the lateral plantar surface of the head of the talus. The anterior and middle facets may form a common, contiguous facet for the talar head and neck.

The posterior tuberosity of the calcaneus [Fig. 3-1 *(B)*] extends posteriorly and downward from the posterior articular facet to form the prominence of the heel. This prominence is visibly absent and difficult to palpate in the clubfoot, because the posterior tuberosity of the calcaneus is pulled upward and inverted by the contracted Achilles tendon. The length and downward inclination of the posterior tuberosity increase the lever arm for the attachment of the tendo Achillis, thereby enhancing its power for push-off.

The Sustentaculum Tali.   This is a horizontal eminence that protrudes upward from the medial border of the calcaneus. This eminence [Fig. 3-1 *(B)*] is an important landmark in understanding the clubfoot deformity and guiding its surgical correction. The sustentaculum is located under the middle articular facet of the calcaneus and, as its name implies, supports the head and neck of the talus. A slip of the tibialis posterior is attached to the sustentaculum tali; in addition, the sustentaculum provides attachments to the deltoid ligament and the plantar calcaneonavicular ligament (spring ligament). It also serves as a pulley for the tendon of the flexor hallucis longus.

The Talus.   Knowledge of the shape of the talus and its articulations is essential for an understanding of the pathomechanics, pathologic anatomy, and treatment of the clubfoot, because the talus undergoes the most changes in form and is also the most susceptible to iatrogenic changes associated with treatment. In the clubfoot, abnormalities in the shape of the talus have a significant affect on the cosmetic and functional end result of correction; therefore, familiarity with the normal contour of the talus is necessary to appreciate the morphologic changes that occur in the clubfoot deformity. The talus, the second largest tarsal bone, is covered with articular cartilage all over except for the small areas of ligamentous attachments. There are no muscle insertions on the talus.

The talus has three parts—a body, a neck, and a head. The body has three articular surfaces collectively known as the *trochlea.* The trochlea articulates with the lower tibia and with the lateral and medial malleoli. It is important to note that the anteroposterior measurement of the superior articular surface of the talus

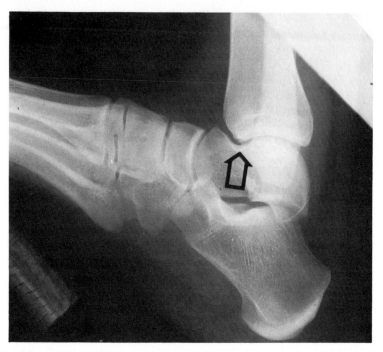

Fig. 3-2. Normal foot held in maximum dorsiflexion. Constriction in the neck of the talus is necessary to allow all of the anterior portion of the trochlea to enter the joint for full dorsiflexion. The posterior half of the trochlea is out of the joint, not in contact with the tibia. The degree of constriction in the neck and the normal range of dorsiflexion are variable.

is greater than the corresponding surface on the lower end of the tibia; this surface is wedge-shaped, being broader anteriorly. Inman[9] has shown that the lateral border of the superior surface and the lateral fibular side of the trochlea are longer than the medial side. For this reason, Inman described: "The trochlea of the talus is rarely if ever a section of a cylinder, but is a section of a frustum of a cone whose apex is directed medially and whose apical angle varies considerably from individual to individual." The posterior aspect of the body of the talus has a groove that directs the course of the flexor hallucis longus medially. The lateral tuberosity of this groove is the larger and serves as an attachment for the posterior talofibular ligament. When this lateral tubercle persists as a separate center of ossification, it is known as the os trigonum. In the young child, this groove is quite shallow. On the inferior surface of the body the large concave facet sits on the dome-shaped posterior facet of the calcaneus. It is essential to appreciate that the long axis of the head and neck is directed slightly medially and downward. However, there is considerable variation in the degree of this medial and downward inclination.

The neck is a constricted narrow portion of the talus located between the body and the head. This constricted part of the talus permits dorsiflexion above the right angle when the anterior portion of the body enters the ankle mortise (Fig. 3-2). The roughened surface of the neck serves as an attachment for the capsules of the ankle and the talonavicular joints, as well as for the anterior talofibular and deltoid ligaments.

Anterior to the neck is the round head of the talus, which is completely covered with articular cartilage and has four articular facets. The distal part of the head articulates with the concave surface of the navicular anteriorly. Close inspection of this anterior articular surface of the head reveals its articular cartilage, which extends obliquely and medially downward and laterally upward. These medial and lateral extensions of the articular surface correspond to the medial and lateral migration of the navicular on the head of the talus during inversion and eversion of the foot. The three plantar facets of the head are slightly flattened areas that articulate with the spring ligament and their counterparts on the calcaneus. The most posterior of these three facets lies just in front of the tarsal sulcus at the junction of the neck and head of the talus. It articulates with the middle facet of the calcaneus, located above the sustentaculum. In front of this facet is another articular facet that rests on the spring ligament. The third facet, which is located slightly lateral and anteriorly, articulates with the anterior facet of the calcaneus (Fig. 3-3).

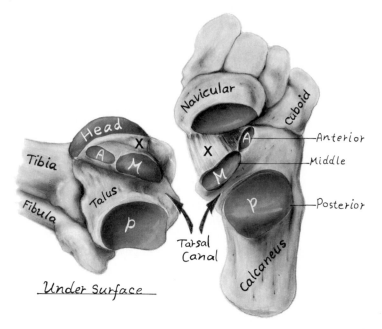

Fig. 3-3.   Talonavicular and subtalar articulations. Anteriorly, the concave surface of the navicular serves as a keystone to support the round head of the talus. "X" marks the site of the spring ligament and the corresponding articular surface of the talus. Additional support for the head of the talus is provided via the anterior and middle subtalar articulations. Posteriorly, the concave undersurface of body of the talus rests on the posterior convex facet of the calcaneus. The tarsal canal separates the subtalar area into anterior and posterior compartments.

The Navicular. This bone is located between the talus and the three cunei-forms. Its posterior surface is concave so as to accomodate and cover the head of the talus. This concavity functions as a keystone to support the head of the talus. The tibialis posterior inserts on the medially prominent tuberosity. The length and proximal extension of the navicular tuberosity is quite variable; in about 2 percent of individuals it persists as an accessory ossicle in the posterior tibial tendon insertion. To date, I have not seen an accessory navicular tuberosity in a patient with a congenital clubfoot deformity.

The Cuboid. This bone has three articular surfaces—anterior, posterior, and medial. Anteriorly it articulates with the fourth and fifth metatarsals; posteriorly it forms a stable S-shaped articulation with the anterior end of the calcaneus; and medially it articulates with the lateral cuneiform. The cuboid is firmly wedged between the bones with which it articulates.

JOINTS OF THE FOOT AND ANKLE

In 1911 Fick[4] recognized the close functional relationship between the foot and ankle when he described the upper ankle joint, art. crurotalaris, and the lower ankle joint, art. talocalcaneal navicularis.

The Tibiotalar Joint. The upper ankle joint is a hinge-like structure. The trochlea of the talus forms a tenon wedged in a mortise formed by the lower tibia and the medial and lateral malleoli. The tibia and fibula are firmly bound together by the tibiofibular interosseous ligaments. Additional stability to the bony mortise is provided by the medial and lateral ligaments of the ankle joint. Vertical motion of the ankle results from an upward and downward gliding movement of the trochlea in the mortise. Since there are no muscle attachments on the talus, its movement is a passive motion that results from the ligamentous attachments and articulations with the calcaneus and the navicular. The talus cannot move alone; it follows the motion of the other bones. Consequently, all motions in the subtalar joints are intimately connected with the vertical motions of the ankle joint. It is important to remember that in full dorsiflexion and plantar flexion only slightly more than half of the dome of the trochlea is in contact with the articular surface of the tibia at any one time. Because the anteroposterior measure-ment of the superior surface of the talus is greater than the reciprocal articular surface of the lower tibia, a portion of the dome of the talus is always out of the mortise and not in contact with the tibia.[9] In plantar flexion, the anterior part of the body is out of the mortise. As a consequence, secondary changes in the shape of this part of the talus can develop in the growing infant when the equinus position is severe and prolonged. In dorsiflexion, the constricted neck of the talus allows all of the anterior portion of the body to enter the mortise (Fig. 3-2). Upward and downward movements of the ankle take place in a slightly oblique axis and not perpendicular to the horizontal. In plantar flexion, the axis of motion is, of necessity, inclined medially, because the lateral border of the trochlea of the talus is longer than the medial side, and because the head and neck of the talus are directed medially relative to the body. In equinus, the head of the talus must move downward and medially, together with the anterior end of the calcaneus, which inverts as the navicular moves medially on the talar head. Vertical motion would be perpendicular (90°) to the horizontal if the trochlea were shaped as a section of a cylinder, with equal medial and lateral borders, and the neck and head were anterior to the body.

Ligaments of the Ankle Joint. *The deltoid ligament.* This strong, dense, fan-shaped structure arises from the medial malleolus and consists of a superficial and deep layer. The superficial portion has three components that run from the tibia to the navicular, to the spring ligament, and to the calcaneus. The deep portion of the deltoid ligament inserts on the neck and the medial surface of the body of the talus. Anatomy texts delineate separate layers of the deltoid ligament; however, the superficial and deep components appear in vivo as one broad mass of ligamentous tissue, which is really a thickened part of the medial capsule closely adherent to the periosteum and tendon sheath of the tibialis posterior in the region of the medial malleolus. The posterior capsule of the ankle can be considered a posterior extension of the deep deltoid, whereas the posterior talocalcaneal ligament is essentially a continuation of the superficial layer of the deltoid.

Whereas medially the deltoid is one continuous structure, the *three lateral ligaments* consist of three separate bands that radiate from the fibula. *The anterior talofibular ligament* runs anteriorly to the neck of the talus. *The calcaneofibular ligament* runs vertically downward to insert on the calcaneus. *The posterior talofibular ligament* is deep-seated and runs medially in a more horizontal plane to attach to an eminence on the posterior body of the talus lateral to the groove for the flexor hallucis longus tendon. The calcaneofibular ligament and the posterior talofibular ligaments are often involved in the pathologic anatomy of the clubfoot, because they are lax in plantar flexion and therefore prone to become contracted in an uninterrupted, persistent equinus position.

Subtalar and Midtarsal Joints. The talus, which is interposed between the tibia above and the calcaneus and navicular below, functions as a saddle between the leg and the foot. During vertical motion in the ankle joint, simultaneous horizontal motions of inversion and eversion are necessary to allow walking on inclines and on uneven terrain; thus the combination of the upper and lower ankle joint motion allows simultaneous motion in two axes, approximately perpendicular to each other.

The subtalar joints. Usually, when orthopedists speak of the subtalar joint they lump the three talocalcaneal articulations together. Anatomically, however, the subtalar area is divided into two separate compartments with separate synovial cavities. *The talocalcaneal interosseous ligament* is the structure that divides the subtalar area into the posterior and anterior subtalar joints. This ligament binds the talus and calcaneus together, adding stability to the subtalar area.

The posterior talocalcaneal joint. This saddle-shaped joint is formed by the concave posterior facet under the body of the talus resting on the convex posterior facet of the calcaneus.

The anterior talocalcaneal joint. The middle and anterior talocalcaneal articulations, between the head and neck of the talus above and the anterior end of the calcaneus below, are included in the anterior talocalcaneal joint.

The midtarsal or Chopart's joints. The midtarsal area consists of two articulations: the talonavicular, which is part of the talocalcaneonavicular joint, and the calcaneocuboid joint. The ball-and-socket talonavicular joint is the most mobile of the intertarsal joints. The S-shaped calcaneocuboid joint and strong ligament attachments firmly stabilize the calcaneocuboid part of the midtarsal area. The cuboid is firmly wedged between the calcaneus and the fourth and fifth metatarsals; therefore it bridges the Chopart and Lisfranc areas. Because of this mosaic anatomic arrangement, the gliding mobility of the cuboid is limited by the navicular and the cuneiforms. For these anatomic reasons, the cuboid moves with the anterior end of the calcaneus and the forefoot, with limited motion at the calcaneocuboid joint.

The mobility of the midtarsal joints may increase when the subtalar joint is fixed, as in a congenital talocalcaneal coalition. This additional mobility, combined with the stress on these joints, causes the degenerative changes in the talonavicular and calcaneocuboid joints in patients with this anomaly.

Naviculocuneiform and Lisfranc joints. Very little gliding motion occurs at the naviculocuneiform articulation. Even less movement takes place in the tarsometatarsal area. The first metatarsal articulates only with the medial cuneiform, has weak ligamentous attachments, and is more mobile. The four lateral metatarsals are firmly attached to each other and to the tarsal bones by strong ligaments and interlocking joints. This anatomic arrangement permits minimal gliding in the Lisfranc region, except for the first metatarsal ray.

The talocalcaneonavicular joint. Because this area is involved in the pathomechanics of all hindfoot and midfoot deformities, an understanding of the anatomy and the mechanics of this joint (Fig. 3-4) is extremely important. The talocalcaneonavicular joint is a complex articulation that includes all articulations between the talar head and the anterior end of the calcaneus, the navicular, and the plantar calcaneonavicular ligament (spring). The posterior talocalcaneal joint is not included; the anterior subtalar and midtarsal joints are included in this complex joint. The talocalcaneonavicular joint has the configuration of a ball-and-socket joint. The acetabulum for the round head of the talus is formed by the posterior concave surfaces of the navicular, the middle and anterior facets of the anterior part of the calcaneus, and the spring ligament.

The *spring ligament* bridges the interval between the navicular and the sustentaculum tali. It has a fibrocartilagenous central part that supports the medial portion of the talar head. Within the posterior subtalar joint, the calcaneal facet is convex and the corresponding talar facet is concave, whereas within the anterior compartment the reverse is true, i.e., the navicular and calcaneal facets form a concave socket for the convex talar head. This alternating convexity and concavity of the infratalar articulations, together with the ligaments that bind the talus to the calcaneus and the navicular, make the subtalar joint quite stable. Because of this anatomic arrangement, subtalar dislocations without fracture are rare.

The composite socket for the head of the talus is completed by fibroelastic tissues that supplement the bony elements noted previously. These structures are arranged as follows: dorsomedially are the talonavicular capsule, the deltoid ligament, and the tendon of the tibialis posterior; subtalarly, the spring ligament;

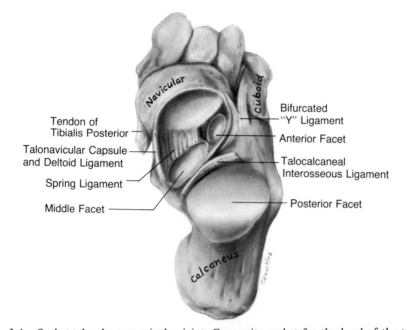

Fig. 3-4.   Socket-talocalcaneonavicular joint. Composite socket for the head of the talus, formed by fibroelastic structures and, in part, bones. Note the large contribution of fibroelastic tissues: below by the important spring ligament, and dorsomedially by the tibialis posterior, deltoid ligament and talonavicular capsule, which blend to form a common mass of elastic tissue. In varus the capacity of the socket is diminished and the elastic components are lax. If these structures are pictured in a relaxed state, the importance of contractures of these soft parts in a clubfoot can be appreciated. In horizontal motions, the above unit moves around the talus, medially with inversion and laterally during eversion. In inversion, the anterior end of the calcaneus angulates medially under the talus, at the same time that the navicular moves medially around the head of the talus closer to the sustentaculum tali. Horizontal motions are limited if the navicular cannot rotate freely around the talar head. The cuboid follows the anterior end of the calcaneus; very little motion occurs at the calcaneocuboid joint.

laterally, the calcaneonavicular portion of the bifurcated or Y ligament; and posteriorly, the talocalcaneal interosseous ligament (Figs. 3-3 and 3-4).

Barclay Smith[13] compared the talocalcaneonavicular joint to the ball-and-socket hip joint. Although it resembles an enarthrodial joint, there are two distinct differences which are very important for the understanding of the pathological anatomy of the clubfoot. In the talocalcaneonavicular joint, the acetabulum moves around the ball, just the opposite from the mechanics of the hip joint. In the hip, the socket is formed by one bone, and the size of its socket is fixed; in contrast, in the talocalcaneonavicular joint two bones and ligaments form a socket that has the capacity to enlarge and diminish in size because it is composed of fibroelastic tissues and two bones that do not articulate with each other. (The navicular and the calcaneus are connected via the spring and Y-ligaments.)

MOVEMENTS OF THE FOOT

Horizontal Motions

Movement at the talonavicular and the anterior and posterior subtalar joints elicits horizontal motions (Fig. 3-4). The anterior end of the calcaneus and the navicular move together in unison around the talar head; most horizontal motion takes place at the talonavicular and the anterior subtalar joints. Less movement occurs in the posterior subtalar joint, and the calcaneocuboid joint has a very limited gliding mobility (the cuboid moves with the calcaneus). For normal subtalar motion, the navicular must be mobile and free to rotate around the talar head. Lapidus[10] has shown that "the heel cannot be everted or inverted without simultaneous motion between the navicular and the head of the talus." Fick [4] and Manter[11] have also demonstrated that movement in the subtalar joint is limited when the talonavicular is transfixed—"when displacement of the navicular is prevented, little movement can be obtained in the subtalar joint." They also showed that "movement in the midtarsal joint was greatly restricted when the subtalar joint was immobilized." These investigators have demonstrated that when displacement of the navicular is prevented, motion in the subtalar joint is limited and vice versa. Restriction of either the talonavicular or subtalar motion affects the mobility of the other; neither functions independently of the other, and in horizontal motion both joints move simultaneously.

Inversion

When the normal foot is adducted and inverted (supination), the navicular rotates medially around the head of the talus, moving proximally and slightly downward and closer to the medial malleolus, thereby diminishing the interval between the navicular and the sustentaculum. At the same time, as the navicular moves medially the calcaneus inverts and lies under the talus. The tibialis posterior—by virtue of its insertion on the navicular, the spring ligament, and the sustentaculum tali of the calcaneus—is the active force that pulls the navicular and the anterior end of the calcaneus medially. This medial migration of the navicular and calcaneus diminishes the size of the acetabulum for the head of the talus, and the sinus tarsi opens laterally.

Medial movement of the navicular and calcaneus during inversion can be demonstrated on the radiograph of a normal foot held in varus and adduction. The x-ray appearance of a normal foot held in the equinovarus position is similar to that of an uncorrected clubfoot [Fig. 3-5(A,B,C)]. This is the reason Scarpa called the clubfoot a congenital subluxation of the talocalcaneonavicular joint,[12] or others consider the deformity a fixed exaggeration of the normal equinovarus position.[1,3] When the foot is inverted, the capacity of the socket is diminished and the lateral part of the talar head is uncovered as a result of the medial and proximal migration of the socket. In this position, the medial and plantar fibroelastic components of the socket are shortened. In the clubfoot, these soft-tissue components of the acetabulum constitute the contractures of the socket, which is smaller

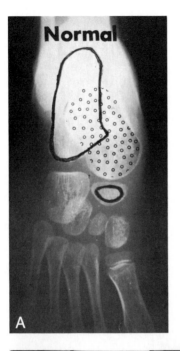

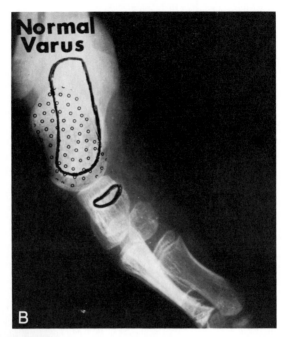

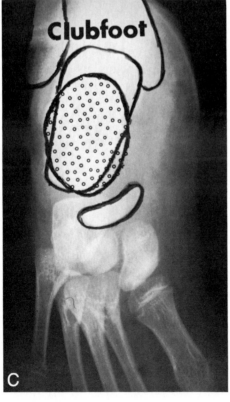

Fig. 3-5. *(A),* Radiograph of a normal foot illustrating the normal relationship of the calcaneus, navicular, and talus. Note the normal divergence between the talus and calcaneus; the navicular is located anterior to the head of the talus. *(B),* The same normal foot forced into inversion. Note the superimposition and diminished divergence of the hindfoot; the navicular is now rotated medially in relation to the head of the talus. *(C),* Clubfoot in a 6-year old child. Note the similarity between this uncorrected clubfoot and the normal foot held in the equinovarus position. The bony prominence over the dorsolateral, common in clubfoot, represents the uncovered head and neck of the talus caused by the medial migration of the navicular and inversion of the calcaneus.

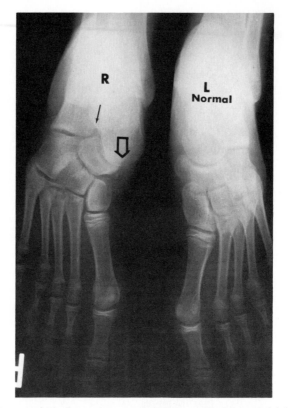

Fig. 3-6. Right congenital planovalgus compared to patient's normal left foot illustrates lateral subluxation of the talocalcaneonavicular socket. Note the lateral angulation of the calcaneus (increased hindfoot divergence) in the right foot accompanied by lateral subluxation of the navicular. The calcaneocuboid relationship remains normal. Clinically, this patient had a bony prominence below the medial malleolus, which was the unexposed medial part of the head of the talus, resulting from eversion of the calcaneus, and lateral subluxation of the navicular with collapse of the arch.

than the normal. Hence, Brockman's definition of a clubfoot as "congenital atresia of the astragalo-calcaneal-scaphoid joint."

Eversion

When the foot is abducted and everted (pronation), movement of the socket is just the opposite of inversion—the calcaneus everts and the navicular moves laterally with the calcaneus in relation to the talus. The capacity of the socket is greater; more of the talar head is covered by the acetabulum, and the sinus tarsi is closed (Fig. 3-6).

Dorsiflexion and Plantar Flexion

Vertical movements of the foot involve motion—not only in the tibiotalar joint but, of necessity, in the talocalcaneonavicular joint as well.[8,10] Because

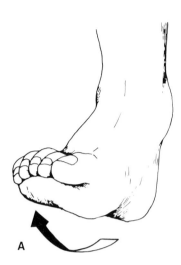

Fig. 3-7. Dorsiflexion. *(A),* In dorsiflexion the foot pronates. *(B),* The calcaneus everts as the navicular moves laterally. *(C),* The talus is horizontal. Only the anterior portion of the trochlea of the talus articulates with the tibia; the posterior part is extraarticular. Relaxation of the triceps permits downward excursion of the posterior tuberosity of the calcaneus, while simultaneous relaxation of the tibialis posterior is necessary to allow upward movement and eversion of the anterior end of the calcaneus. The degree of dorsiflexion gradually lessens with maturity.

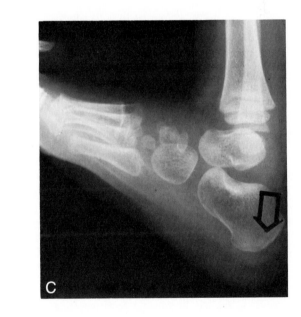

the talus has no muscle attachments, it cannot move alone; it must follow the motions of the calcaneus and the navicular.

Dorsiflexion [Fig. 3-7 *(A,B,C)*] of the tibiotalar joint is accompanied by pronation of the foot. Upward movement of the foot requires simultaneous relaxation of the triceps and the tibialis posterior to permit a downward migration of the posterior tuberosity of the calcaneus as the anterior end of the calcaneus everts while the navicular moves laterally on the talus.

In plantar flexion [Fig. 3-8 *(A,B,C)*], the foot supinates. Downward motion of the foot is a combination of equinus, inversion, and adduction. In plantar flexion, the tibialis posterior pulls the navicular medially, and inverts and pulls the anterior

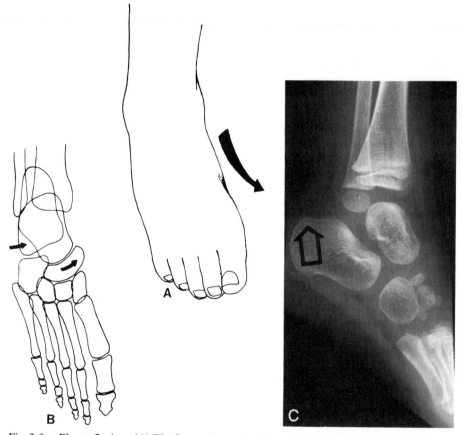

Fig. 3-8.   Plantarflexion. *(A)*, The foot supinates in plantarflexion. *(B)*, The calcaneus inverts as the navicular moves medially. *(C)*, The talus is in a vertical position. Notice the anterior half of the trochlea of the talus is out of the mortise while its posterior portion is in contact with the tibia. In varus, the sinus tarsi is open. The posterior tuberosity of the calcaneus is pulled upward by the tendo Achillis and the tibialis posterior pulls the anterior end downward and medially.

end of the calcaneus downward, via its attachment to the sustentaculum. At the same time, the triceps surae pulls the posterior tuberosity of the calcaneus upward. The triceps and the tibialis posterior are the only extrinsic muscles that insert on the calcaneus. Since they both plantar flex and invert the heel, equinus, varus, and adduction take place simultaneously and not as separate isolated movements of the foot. One can demonstrate this by trying to invert one's own foot; automatically the foot will become adducted and plantar flexed. Eversion is associated with simultaneous abduction and dorsiflexion.

Full dorsiflexion and plantar flexion are not possible without motion in the talocalcaneonavicular complex. Knowledge of the normal mechanics of the equinovarus position should influence our treatment of clubfoot when attempting to correct the equinus and varus components separately. Participation of the talocalcaneonavicular joint in vertical motion of the foot is demonstrated by the peroneal spastic flatfoot, where plantar flexion is limited because inversion is impossible. In contrast, dorsiflexion is usually normal or slightly increased. In an ankle fusion, the slight vertical jog of motion is primarily due to the development of compensatory hyper-mobility in the talocalcaneonavicular complex.

Adduction-Abduction of the Forefoot

In horizontal movements, the forefoot follows the hindfoot, and additional adduction and abduction motions occur at the Lisfranc area, supplementing the motion in the talocalcaneonavicular complex.

REFERENCES

1. Brockman, E. P.: Congenital Clubfoot. John Wright and Sons, Bristol, 1930.
2. Cunningham, D. J.: Textbook of Anatomy. William Wood and Co., New York, 1927.
3. Elmsie, R. C.: Principles in treatment of congenital talipes equinovarus. Journal of Orthopedic Surgery, 2:669, 1920.
4. Fick, R.: Handbuch der Anatomie und Mechanik der Gelenke. Iena, 1911 in Handbachs der Anatomie des Menchen, Zweiter Band. Erste Abteilung, Dritter Teil, p. 626.
5. Grant, J. C. B.: Atlas of Anatomy. Williams and Wilkins, Baltimore, 1962.
6. Gray, H.: Anatomy of the Human Body. Lea and Febiger, Philadelphia, 1959.
7. Henry, A. K.: Extensive Exposure applied to Limb Surgery. Williams and Wilkins, Baltimore, 1946.
8. Hicks, J. H.: Mechanics of the foot. Journal of Anatomy, *87*, 1953.
9. Inman, V. T.: The Joints of the Ankle. Williams and Wilkins, Baltimore, 1976.
10. Lapidus, P. W.: Subtalar joint, its anatomy and mechanics. Bulletin of the Hospital for Joint Diseases, *16*, 1955.
11. Manter, J. T.: Movements of the Subtalar and Transverse Tarsal Joints. The Anatomical Record, *80*, 1941.
12. Scarpa, A.: A memoir on the congenital clubfeet of children. (Translated by J. W. Wishart.) Constable, Edinburgh, 1818.
13. Smith, B.: Journal of Anatomy and Physiology, *30*:390, 1895.

4 | Pathologic Anatomy

Scarpa[13] was one of the first to publish a vivid description of the pathologic anatomy of the clubfoot. He believed that the deformity resulted from an abnormal relationship between the tarsal bones, associated with soft-tissue contractures. He described the "twisting" of the calcaneus and the navicular around the talus as a "congenital dislocation of the talocalcaneonavicular joint." Adams,[1] in 1866, described essentially the same abnormalities in his classic work, *The Clubfoot, Its Causes, Pathology and Treatment.* Adams called attention to the abnormal shape of the head and neck of the talus, which he felt were secondarily acquired deformities. Bissell,[3] in 1888, also noted the talar deformity but believed that the altered shape of the talus represented a primary bony distortion. Brockman,[5] in 1930, stated that these abnormalities were the result of a "congenital atresia" of the socket that contains the head of the talus. Brockman and other investigators[6] have compared the clubfoot to the normal equinovarus position and described the deformity as a fixed exaggeration of the normal equinovarus position. Since 1803, most investigators have reported essentially the same abnormal anatomy as was initially described by Scarpa and Adams.

The literature[14,18] describing dissections of clubfeet also reveals that most authors agree with the concept outlined by Scarpa and Adams. Investigators have continued to describe the same morphologic changes in the talus, while emphasizing slight variations in other aspects of the pathology. The apparent differences of opinion suggest a difference in semantics rather than any disagreement regarding the basic pathology of clubfoot. Hence, while there is much disagreement regarding the cause and treatment of clubfoot, except for some minor variations, most investigators have generally agreed on the major basic underlying abnormality.

I do not mean to imply that all investigators subscribed to Scarpa's concept. Some authors[8] have maintained that the primary abnormality is an inward or outward rotation of the talus in the ankle mortise. Another concept is that the essential abnormality lies in the midtarsal joints;[7] and that the other elements of the deformity, including the heel varus, are secondary adaptive changes. (The

35

inward deviation at the midtarsal joints results in a lengthening of the lateral border of the foot.) Attenborough[2] states: "The fundamental deformity is a plantar flexed talus." Most investigators, including myself, have adopted the concept reported by Scarpa and Adams.

REASONS FOR DIVERGENT OPINIONS

Many factors are responsible for the disagreement regarding concepts of the pathologic anatomy of clubfoot. A major reason for the disagreement has been the failure to differentiate idiopathic clubfoot from the deformity associated with multiple congenital anomalies. Since many conditions can cause talipes equinovarus, it is not surprising that the abnormalities will vary and will not be consistently the same in all feet. Another reason for the differing hypotheses is the inability or failure to distinguish secondary adapted changes from primary defects, especially the failure to appreciate that all the pathology evident at birth is not necessarily primary (changes may be acquired secondarily during intrauterine development of the fetus). Further disagreement has occurred because most dissections have been done on premature fetuses born with a clubfoot that is a local manifestation of a systemic syndrome, a neurologic disorder, or multiple congenital anomalies. Very few dissections have been carried out on true idiopathic clubfeet. Many of the specimens had spinal cord defects, which are notorious for their variability.

MATERIALS AND METHODS

This discussion will be limited to the pathologic anatomy of the idiopathic clubfoot—i.e., when the foot deformity is the only congenital defect. For the most part, this study is based on the correlation of clinical and radiographic examinations with the abnormal anatomy found in a large series of clubfoot operations. I have also had the opportunity to dissect one untreated idiopathic clubfoot of an otherwise normal, full-term baby who died in infancy from an unrelated infection.* Significant information was also obtained from surgical experiences with a small series of children, 16 months to 5 years of age, who had had no prior treatment; this work provided an opportunity to observe the natural course of this congenital defect unaltered by any form of therapy. In addition to the contributions by Scarpa,[13] Adams,[1] Bissell,[3] and Brockman,[5] studies by many other investigators have provided additional sources of information on the pathologic anatomy of clubfoot.

Abnormal Findings Vary.   Through the years I have been impressed that the pathologic anatomy noted at surgery, the clinical features, and the radiographic appearance of the abnormality will vary in each case, depending on the severity of the deformity, the age of the patient, and prior treatment. The basic pathology is essentially the same, however, and some consistent abnormalities are found in all cases of clubfoot. The differences are variations in the degree of deformity,

---

* Courtesy of Professor R. T. Domenech, Universidade Federal Da Bahia, Salvador, Brasil.

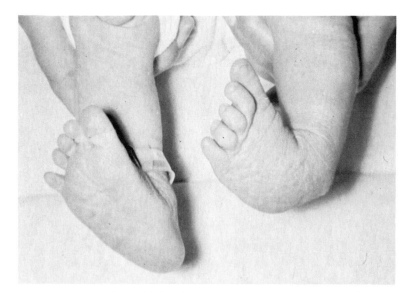

Fig. 4-1. Left clubfoot. Typical left talipes equinovarus in newborn. Notice dorsiflexion in normal right foot.

the clinical appearance, and minor additional or absent abnormalities that were noted in the pathologic anatomy at surgery.

The following discussion of the morbid anatomy will include the abnormalities I observed. However, it must be emphasized that all clubfeet do not necessarily have all of the abnormal variations to be described. Even bilateral deformities are not identical. There are slight differences in the clinical appearance and pathologic findings; one foot is usually more resistant and deformed than the other. In bilateral deformities the more resistant foot may be either the right or the left; laterality does not appear to be related to a right-handed surgeon applying more effective manipulation and plaster immobilization on the patient's right foot.

The Deformity

Talipes. Initially, the term clubfoot was applied indiscriminately to all deformed feet. In 1839, however, Little[11] proposed the generic term talipes—derived from the latin *talus* (ankle) and *pes* (foot)—to describe all foot deformities, stating: "I have proposed to employ the classical word *talipes,* as a generic term, to include all those deformities of the feet produced by contraction of certain muscles: and to use the terms varus, valgus, and equinus to designate the specific forms of these diseases." Thus clubfoot became *talipes equinovarus,* a definition that is universally accepted and clearly describes a deformity of equinus and varus.

Clinical Features. The typical clubfoot consists of a deformed foot in equinus, varus, adduction, and, in some cases, a cavus component (Fig. 4-1). Varying degrees of deformity can be seen in the newborn. The deformity may be mild and appear to be only a slight exaggeration of the normal equinovarus position, or it may be

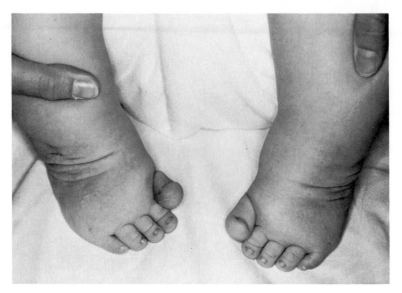

Fig. 4-2.   Rigid clubfeet. Feet are short, stubby. Note foreshortened first metatarsal ray.

so severe that the foot lies almost in contact with the medial boarder of the tibia. In addition to variations in the severity of the deformity, the degree of associated rigidity also varies. Some feet are extremely rigid and very little change is visible after manipulation. These are usually smaller, stubby feet with a shortened first metatarsal ray (Fig. 4-2). Feet that are less rigid and more pliable on manipulation are usually a little longer than those with rigid deformities (Fig. 4-3).

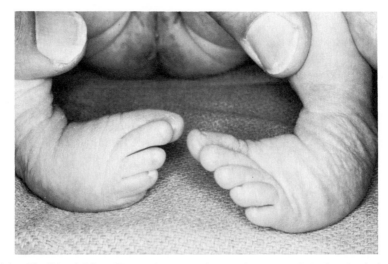

Fig. 4-3.   Flexible clubfeet. Feet and toes are longer than normal. Deformity is less rigid on manipulation.

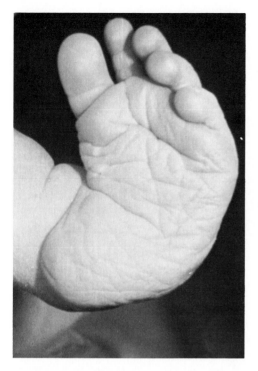

Fig. 4-4. Left clubfoot. Inversion of heel is accompanied by adduction and varus of the forefoot. *Note:* medial border of foot is concave and elevated.

Deformities that can be almost fully corrected on initial manipulation should not be considered true idiopathic congenital clubfeet, but rather mild positional deformities. These are deformities that are usually corrected completely after 4 to 6 weeks of treatment with manipulation and plaster immobilization, passive stretching, or tarsopronator shoes attached to a Denis Browne bar. In my opinion, this latter group and metatarsus adductus should not be included in a study of idiopathic clubfeet.

Equinus deformity of the foot is accompanied by an inversion of the heel, adduction, and varus of the forefoot. The medial border of the foot is concave and elevated, and its plantar surface faces upward; the lateral border of the foot is convex and depressed downward. The posterior tuberosity of the heel is pulled upward, inverted, difficult to palpate, and less visible (Fig. 4-4). The older child may have a callous on the dorsal aspect of the fifth metatarsal. The bony prominence visible and palpable over the dorsal lateral aspect of the foot represents the head and neck of the talus, which are partially uncovered because the navicular and the calcaneus have been displaced medially [(Fig. 4-5 *(A, B)*].

Skin Abnormalities

Changes in the appearance of the skin are quite variable. The skin over the dorsolateral aspect of the foot is usually stretched out, thin, and atrophied; rarely, there is a mild abrasion in this area at birth. Some feet have a deep cleft on the medial plantar surface; usually they have a severe cavus component with a forefoot

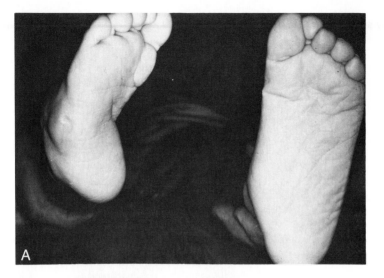

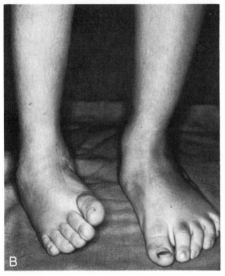

Fig. 4-5.   Uncorrected right clubfoot in a 4-year-old child. *(A)*, Callus on dorsal aspect of fifth metatarsal secondary to weight bearing on deformed inverted foot. *(B)*, Note bony prominence (head and neck of talus) anterior to lateral malleolus, compared to normal left foot.

flexion contracture that contributes to the equinus deformity (Fig. 4-6). Some feet that are rigid and have a severe equinovarus deformity also have a single deep cleft in the skin just above the heel; the prominence of the heel is even more obscured in these deformities (Fig. 4-7). The skin along the medial aspect of the foot below the medial malleolus is contracted and "notoriously poorly nourished,"[12] an important consideration in surgical treatment.

PATHOGNOMONIC SIGNS OF IDIOPATHIC CLUBFOOT

In the normal newborn, the foot is extremely pliable and hypermobile; on passive dorsiflexion, the dorsum of the foot will usually touch or closely approximate

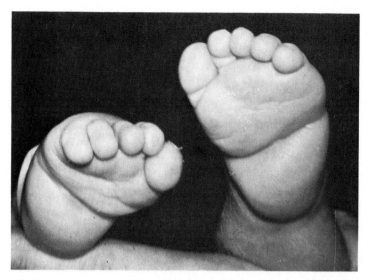

Fig. 4-6.   Clubfeet with deep plantar clefts. Deep cleft in skin associated with forefoot flexion contributes to composite equinus deformity.

the anterior aspect of the lower tibia. In the clubfoot, dorsiflexion is impossible, and even when strong pressure is applied the foot remains in the equinovarus position. The normal foot has skin creases in the region of the Achilles insertion on the posterior tuberosity of the calcaneus, whereas the skin in this area of the clubfoot is smooth and the usual wrinkles are absent. A plausable explanation for the absent skin creases in the region of the heel is that the fixed equinus deformity prevented the normal upward and downward excursion of the posterior

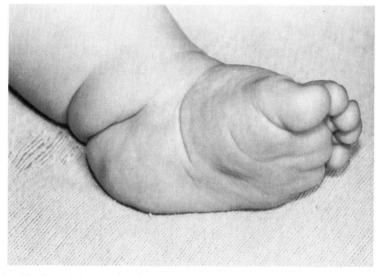

Fig. 4-7.   Clubfoot with deep cleft just above heel. The posterior tuberosity of the calcaneus, which is pulled upward and inverted, is difficult to see or palpate.

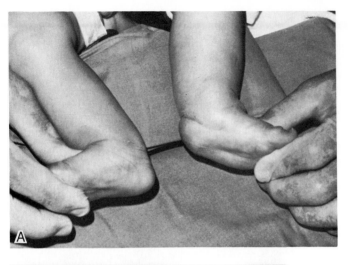

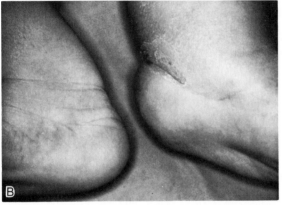

Fig. 4-8. Clubfoot in a 3-month-old infant. *(A),* Passive dorsiflexion on the normal right. The posterior tuberosity is prominent and moves downward. In the clubfoot, the posterior tuberosity stays upward and inverted. *(B),* A close-up view demonstrates absent skin creases in the clubfoot, compared to the normal right foot.

tuberosity of the calcaneus. Hence, the skin remained contracted and was never alternately stretched and relaxed, as in the normal vertical motions of the posterior tuberosity [Fig. 4-8 *(A, B)*]. In my experience, patients who have an equinus deformity and skin creases in this area of the heel do not have true congenital clubfeet. Rather, the deformity is acquired and nonidiopathic, as in a muscular dystrophy, or a positional deformity.

The Knee and Lower Leg

At birth, the knee joint appears normal, with the usual knee flexion contracture seen in the newborn. A hyperextension deformity becomes evident later, after the child begins walking. Back knee, or hyperextension of the knee joint, develops as a consequence of the fixed equinus deformity of the foot. The elongated posterior structures of the knee usually regain their normal length after the foot deformity is corrected. Usually, at birth atrophy of the lower leg is not a prominent feature; the discrepancy in the size of the calf becomes more evident as the child grows. Genuvalgum is common in the older child with a severe, uncorrected bilateral equinovarus deformity; this is a compensatory acquired adaptation as the child attempts to place the more deformed foot in a plantigrade position. The valgus deformity of the knee usually occurs on the side that is more severely deformed and is usually associated with considerable external rotation of the ankle joint (Fig. 4-9).

The Tibia

Much has been written for and against the existence of tibia vara and internal tibial torsion in the clubfoot deformity. I believe the significance of tibia vara has been overemphasized; the basic pathology lies in the foot, with adaptive changes in the leg. Many children with clubfeet also have varying degrees of tibia vara that is no greater than that seen in children without clubfeet. In the past, internal tibial torsion has been incriminated as a cause of recurrent deformity. However, failures of external derotational osteotomy operations are evidence that this is a misconception.

The Ankle

In the normal foot, the ankle mortise faces slightly laterally. In the clubfoot, this external rotation of the mortise is increased.[2,10,16] In resistant feet, this lateral

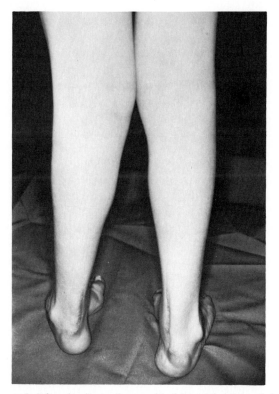

Fig. 4-9. Uncorrected deformity in an 8-year-old child with bilateral deformity who had two unsuccessful soft-tissue operations on each foot. Note genuvalgum on the more severely deformed left side.

orientation of the tibiofibular unit increases with age. Some of the increased lateral rotation may be acquired as a result of repeated attempts to dorsiflex and evert the foot when the rigid contractures do not stretch. The ankle may yield to this external rotating force by rotating laterally. Another factor is the child's attempt to compensate for the varus adduction deformity of the foot by rotating the leg externally on weight bearing and walking. The lateral malleolus is palpable posteriorly, which is to be expected with the increased external rotation of the mortise. The medial malleolus is usually underdeveloped and appears to be slightly anterior to its normal position. In addition to the abnormal lateral orientation of the ankle joint, the relationship of the diaphyses of the tibia and fibula is abnormal. I have noticed while performing a tibialis posterior muscle transfer through the interosseous space in a clubfooted child that the distance between the tibia and fibula is markedly diminished in comparison to a normal leg. The reason for this is obscure, but one may hypothesize that it is related to the exaggerated lateral rotation of the tibia and fibula at the ankle joint.

PATHOLOGIC ANATOMY OF CLUBFOOT

Having reviewed the normal anatomy and mechanics of the foot and ankle, I will now discuss the abnormal anatomy of the clubfoot. As previously stated, an understanding of this morbid anatomy and an appreciation of its deviation from the normal are essential in order to formulate a rational method of treatment that will fulfill the goal of restoring normal anatomy and normal function to the foot.[17,18]

The clubfoot deformity is due to the abnormal relationship of the tarsal bones; the navicular and calcaneus are displaced medially around the talus (Fig. 4-10). Correction of this abnormal tarsal relationship is resisted or prevented by pathologic contractures of the associated soft parts. The severity of the deformity depends upon the degree of bony displacement, whereas the resistance to treatment is determined by the rigidity of soft-tissue contractures. Some of the abnormalities in the bones and soft tissues are acquired as a result of the persistent deformity. The adapted alterations in the shape of the tarsal bones are acquired in accordance with Wolff's law: "Every change in the use of static function of bone causes a change in the internal form and architecture as well as alteration in its external formation and function according to mathematical law." The soft-tissue contractures are acquired in accordance with the law of Davis: "When ligaments and soft tissues are in a loose or lax state they gradually will shorten."

Components of the Deformity

It is customary to divide the clubfoot into separate components: equinus, varus, and adduction, and frequently an associated cavus deformity. Anatomically, equinus, varus, and adduction should be considered composites of deformities which include abnormalities in the ankle, subtalar, midtarsal joints, and the forefoot.

Equinus. The foot is fixed in the plantar-flexed position. As noted in the discussion of normal mechanics in plantar flexion, both the ankle and the talocalcaneonavicular joints are involved, and, in addition, the plantar-flexion deformity

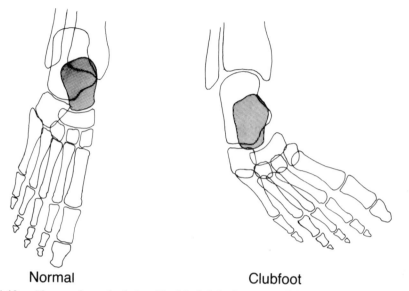

Normal   Clubfoot

Fig. 4-10.   Abnormal tarsal relationship. Medial displacement of the calcaneus and navicular around the talus. Note the cuboid and the forefoot accompanying the hindfoot.

of the forefoot may also contribute to this component of the deformity. Equinus deformity is a composite of ankle joint equinus, inversion of the talocalcaneonavicular complex, and plantar flexion of the forefoot.

Varus.   The hindfoot is rotated inward. This occurs primarily in the talocalcaneonavicular joint. The whole tarsus, with the exception of the talus, is rotated inward with respect to the lower leg. Since the forefoot follows the inverted hindfoot, its medial border faces upward, thereby contributing to the composite varus deformity.

Adduction.   The foot is rotated inward. This medial displacement occurs at the talonavicular and the anterior subtalar joint. In addition, some medial deviation occurs at the tarsometatarsal area and contributes to this part of the deformity. The first metatarsal usually appears shorter; the big toe is short, stubby, and wider than normal.

Cavus.   The forefoot plantar flexion, which Brockman described as a plantaris, causes a cavus deformity and also contributes to the composite equinus.

The degree to which any one of these components contributes to the deformity varies with each patient. The equinus, varus, and adduction components are intimately associated with each other. Together they produce the clubfoot deformity, but they are not three separate, isolated elements of deformity. For this reason, as will be demonstrated later, the complete correction of any one component requires simultaneous correction of the other two.

Osseous Deformities

Many investigators have observed that the overall size of all tarsal bones is smaller in the clubfoot than in the normal foot, thus producing an asymmetric size in a unilateral deformity. Both legs are usually equal in length.

The Talus.   While the talus is the least displaced, it undergoes the most severe and consistent changes in form. The talus has no muscle attachments and is passively forced into equinus by its articulations and attachments to the calcaneus and navicular. In the lateral radiograph, it may appear to be extruded or subluxed anteriorly out of the ankle joint.[17]

Body of the talus.   The body of the talus is stabilized by the bony mortise. The application of our knowledge of the normal anatomy of the tibiotalar joint combined with Wolff's law helps us to understand the reason adaptive changes develop in the body of the talus. In the equinus position, only the posterior half of the trochlea articulates with the tibia; the forward portion of the trochlea is out of the mortise anteriorly. One should bear in mind that in a clubfoot the anterior wider part of the body probably never entered the ankle joint; therefore, this portion of the trochlea never had an opportunity to respond to physiologic stress. As a consequence, the anterior trochlea is prone to develop the adaptive morphologic changes noted by Schlicht[14] and others, including the author.

Schlicht dissected eight idiopathic clubfeet and found that the posterior surface of the trochlea was in the mortise and had a normal rounded contour. The anterior half, however, failed to develop a normal configuration. Schlicht observed that the anterior portion of the trochlea

> "was relatively broader than that of the normal foot, and this broadness was further accentuated by the outward flaring of the facet which articulates with the fibula. As a result the superior surface of the talus could not be fully accomodated by the tibio-fibula mortise. Dorsiflexion was resisted by the mortise; this bony block was the most important cause of the persisting equinus deformity."

Neck of the talus.   The most important constant distortion is found in the neck and head of the talus. Normally, the long axis of the neck and head of the talus is directed slightly medially in relation to the body (about 150°). In the clubfoot, this medial deviation of the neck and head is increased to form a more acute angle with the axis of the talar body; the degree of medial inclination is quite variable (115° to 135°; Fig. 4-11). Irani and Sherman[9] are of the opinion that the deformity of the head and neck of the talus represents a *prime germ plasm defect.* There are others who believe that changes in the shape of the anterior part of the talus represent a physiologic response to abnormal articulations with other bones.[1] In addition to increased medial deviation, the neck is foreshortened and the usual constriction of the neck is absent. I have repeatedly observed, especially in the older child, the absence of an identifiable constricted neck, medial deviation of the neck, and an overdeveloped anterior portion of the trochlea, which are more pronounced and readily evident. This heaping-up of bone in this part of the trochlea and neck of the talus, plus the medial deviation of the neck, form a bony mass that impinges on the anterior lip of the tibia in dorsiflexion; thus the entrance of the talus into the mortise is impeded, contributing to the equinus deformity. These abnormalities in the form of the talus are well demonstrated in the uncorrected clubfoot at skeletal maturity. In my experience, the talus has

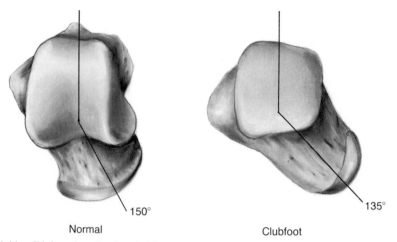

150° Normal   135° Clubfoot

Fig. 4-11.   Right talus. In the clubfoot, the medial deviation of the neck and head of the talus is increased. Note the lack of constriction in the neck associated with overgrowth of the anterior trochlea. In the clubfoot, the talus is smaller and the usual longer lateral border and the wider anterior portion of the trochlea are exaggerated.

shown a considerable capacity to remold in response to normal function after the abnormal tarsal relationship is corrected.

Head of the talus. The round head of the talus normally faces forward and is covered by the concave surface of the navicular. In the clubfoot, the head of the talus and the facet for the navicular face mediad. The talonavicular articulation is oriented in a more sagittal plane compared to the normal coronal orientation. The head of the talus is usually broader than normal, with varying degrees of distortion (flattening). In severe deformities, the head may be almost wedge shaped, with a broad flat surface facing mediad. Correlating the talar head deformity (noted at surgery) with prior treatment suggests that some of the distortion may be attributed to iatrogenic compression of the cartilagenous anlage by manipulative treatment largely because the severity of the deformity was often commensurate with the duration of treatment and the force of the manipulations. Surgical experience with the series of patients who had received no prior treatment whatsoever supports this hypothesis regarding iatrogenic changes to the talar head. In this group of patients with therapeutically virgin feet, the usual increased medial angulation of the head and neck of the talus was present. However, in spite of severe clinical deformities, the head of the talus was rather well preserved and rounded, without the degree of flattening, widening, and foreshortening often found in feet that had received vigorous and prolonged forceful manipulations.

Inferior surface of the talus. The posterior concave facet of the body is less well-developed and more shallow. The three plantar facets of the head usually appear as one contiguous flat surface. The medial borders of the talus and the calcaneus are congruent, oblique, and underdeveloped. I believe this abnormality is secondary to the constant compression of these adjacent surfaces in the fixed varus position.

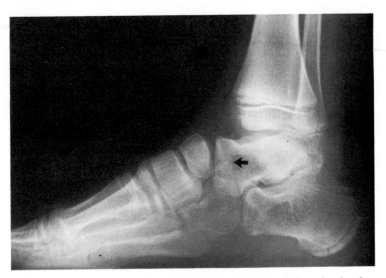

Fig. 4-12.   Secondary changes in talus. The abnormal shape of the talar head can result from forceful compression of manipulation. Note the incongruity of the anterior tibiotalar joint, which was the cause of pain in ankle joint, anteriorly.

The talus at skeletal maturity.   Initially, the major primary deformity is in the head and neck of the talus; too often there is a tendency to overlook the adaptive changes that develop in the anterior portion of the body (Fig. 4-12). At skeletal maturity, the deformity of the trochlea is a cause of pain and problems

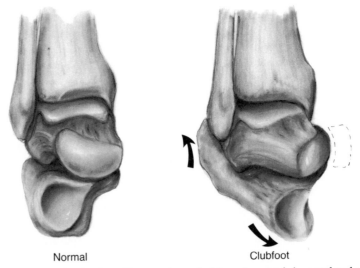

Normal   Clubfoot

Fig. 4-13.   Calcaneus in clubfoot. The anterior end of the calcaneus is inverted and adducted, while the posterior end is displaced upward. Note the calcaneus is in equinus, adducted, and inverted.

in the ankle joint that often compromise the result of a triple arthrodesis, or may even necessitate a pantalar arthrodesis as a salvage procedure.

The Calcaneus. It is important to note that the calcaneus is involved in all three components of the deformity—i.e., equinus, varus, and adduction.[17] The posterior tuberosity is displaced upwards and laterally, while the anterior end is displaced downward, medially, and inverted under the head of the talus (Fig. 4-13). In general, the normal shape is maintained except for changes that occur in the articular surfaces and in the region of the sustentaculum tali. Even in the severely deformed foot, the calcaneus does not exhibit the distortions seen in the talus; the clinical deformity of the heel is due to its abnormal position rather than to an abnormal shape of the bone.

The sustentaculum tali is displaced medially from its normal location under the head of the talus. Not unusually, it is found to be underdeveloped. When the sustentaculum is markedly underdeveloped, it may, following the surgical correction, fail to provide the usual pulley for the flexor hallucis longus, which then tends to fall into the subtalar joint. In some of the very severe deformities in which the heel is markedly inverted, the sustentaculum tali may be adjacent to the head of the talus and much closer to the medial malleolus [Fig. 4-14 *(ABC)*]. The medial articular surface of the calcaneus is underdeveloped and congruent with the corresponding articular surface of the talus; the subtalar joint is slanted more than normal. The posterior convex facet, like its counterpart on the body of the talus, is also underdeveloped. The anterior and middle facets are usually one flat continuous articular surface rather than separate concave well-delineated facets.

The Navicular. The articular surface of the navicular faces medially to articulate with the medially deviated head and neck of the talus. At surgery, I repeatedly found varying degrees of medial displacement of the navicular superimposed on the neck deformity; the navicular may even articulate with the medial malleolus in very severe deformities. On rare occasions the navicular may be subluxed slightly, dorsally and medially; this occurs after prolonged vigorous manipulations. The normal concavity of the proximal articular surface of the navicular is absent, as this surface conforms to the flattened deformed talar head. The navicular tuberosity and the sustentaculum tali are in close proximity to the medial malleolus as a result of the medial displacement of the navicular and varus adduction of the calcaneus. In the older child, the tuberosity of the navicular is usually elongated. The bean-shaped deformity, characterized by a concavity of the medial border of the foot and a convex lateral border, is the result of: (1) varus and adduction of the heel, (2) medial displacement of the navicular on the medially angulated head and neck of the talus, and (3) forefoot adduction (Fig. 4-15).

The Cuboid. Opinions differ regarding the degree of cuboid involvement. Some investigators emphasize significant medial displacement of the cuboid; others, including myself, feel that, while there are some changes at the calcaneocuboid joint, these are minimal when compared to the displacement of the calcaneus and the navicular. The lateral convexity of the foot is predominantly the result of the cuboid moving with the anterior end of the calcaneus, rather than the result of a significant medial displacement of the cuboid relative to the calcaneus.

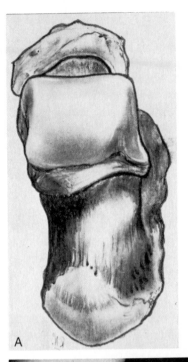

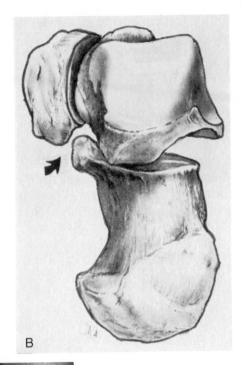

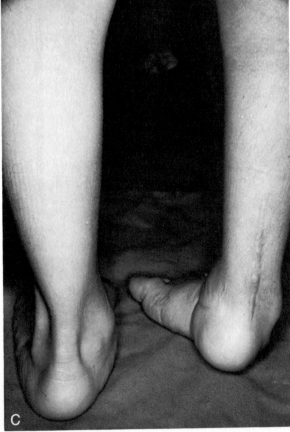

Fig. 4-14. Right calcaneus displacement, rear view. (A), Normal position of calcaneus under the talus; navicular is in front of the talus. (B), This view illustrates the abnormal relationship found at surgery of child shown in (C). The calcaneus is inverted, the sustentaculum tali, with the navicular, are in close approximation with each other and to the medial malleolus. (C), Photograph of 4-year-old boy whose foot demonstrated the pathologic anatomy noted in (B) (A and B reproduced from Fripp, A. T., Shaw, N. E.: Clubfoot. E. & S. Livingstone, Edinburgh and London, 1967.)

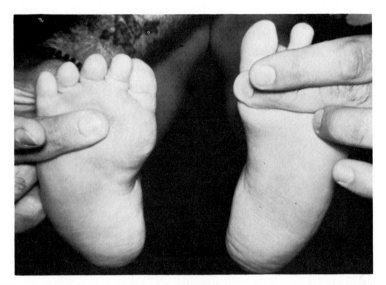

Fig. 4-15. Typical bean-shaped deformity. Medial concavity due to adduction and inversion of the calcaneus with medial displacement of navicular and forefoot adduction.

The proximal end of the cuboid participates in the midtarsal joint (Chopart), and the distal end is part of the tarsometatarsal (Lisfranc) joints. Thus, the cuboid bridges the midtarsal and tarsometatarsal areas. Because of this anatomic relationship, significant medial displacement of the cuboid is obstructed by the navicular and the cuneiforms.

I have also noticed (when performing a triple arthrodesis for an uncorrected clubfoot) that unlike the displacement at the talonavicular joint, no appreciable deformity is present in the calcaneocuboid joint. This observation provides evidence that changes in the calcaneocuboid joint are minimal in the clubfoot. Additional corroborative evidence is provided by my experience with surgically correcting clubfeet without mobilizing the calcaneocuboid joint.

The Cuneiforms and Metatarsals. The cuneiforms show minimal changes and the metatarsals even less. The medial migration and inversion of all five metatarsals cause the forefoot adduction that contributes to the convexity of the lateral border of the foot and the composite varus adduction deformity. Plantar flexion of the forefoot on the hindfoot contributes to the composite equinus deformity and cavus.

Soft-Tissue Contractures

The soft-tissue contractures include the muscles, tendons, tendon sheaths, ligaments, joint capsules, and skin. In the severe equinus deformity, it is well to bear in mind that the posterior tibial neurovascular bundle may also be shortened. Contractures of the soft parts conform to the abnormal tarsal relationship and are as variable as the bony distortion.

The degree of shortening varies; the same contractures are not present in all

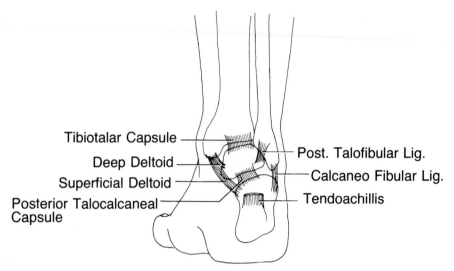

Tibiotalar Capsule

Deep Deltoid

Superficial Deltoid

Posterior Talocalcaneal
Capsule

Post. Talofibular Lig.

Calcaneo Fibular Lig.

Tendoachillis

Fig. 4-16.   Posterior contractures.

cases to the same degree. For example, in some patients the tendon sheaths are very dense and contracted, while in others the tendon sheaths contribute very little to the resistance. On occasion, even the posterior capsule of the ankle joint may be almost normal. Fibrosis and scar tissue are always more severe following previous surgery. I have noticed that contractures usually are denser and more shortened in children who have had little or no prior treatment; collagen contractures also appear to be more dense and thickened in blacks and mulattoes. While there are variations between patients, some constant, soft-tissue contractures are present in all cases. The Achilles tendon, tibialis posterior, deltoid, spring ligaments, and the talonavicular capsule are prime contractures common to all patients. To correlate pathology with the components of the deformity, contractures are divided into the following four groups: posterior, medial plantar, subtalar, and plantar.

Posterior Contractures. *(Tendo Achillis, tibiotalar capsule, talocalcaneal capsule, posterior talofibular ligament, calcaneofibular ligament)*

Posterior contractures (Fig. 4-16) resist correction of the equinus deformity of the ankle joint and the calcaneus. The posterior capsules of the tibiotalar and the talocalcaneal joints are shortened. Of the two, the posterior capsule of the talocalcaneal articulation is usually more contracted and the more important. Occasionally, especially in younger children with milder deformities, the capsule of the tibiotalar joint may have almost normal elasticity or a mild contracture. The Achilles tendon is always contracted, and the amount of shortening is quite variable. In the clubfoot, the Achilles attachment is broader and it inserts more distally on the medial surface of the calcaneus, thereby contributing to the heel varus. This abnormal insertion is an adaptive change that occurs because the tendon attaches itself to the deviated posterior end of the calcaneus. In the older child, the posterior talofibular and the calcaneofibular ligaments may also be contracted.

The contracted Achilles, posterior talocalcaneal ligament, and the calcaneofibular ligament are the structures that resist correction of the equinus deformity of the calcaneus. These contracted structures prevent the downward excursion of the posterior tuberosity of the calcaneus, which is necessary for dorsiflexion. The shortened posterior capsule of the ankle joint and the posterior talofibular ligament are contractures that resist dorsiflexion of the talus; they prevent the downward exit of the back portion of the trochlea out of the mortise, a prerequisite for dorsiflexion. Elmslie[6] and later Bost[4] called attention to the upward and outward displacement of the posterior tuberosity of the calcaneus, and established the rationale for sectioning the calcaneofibular ligament.

Medial Plantar Contractures. *(Tibialis posterior tendon, deltoid ligament, talonavicular capsule, and spring ligament)*

Medial plantar contractures (Fig. 4-17) are the most important and resistant in the clubfoot. They include the tibialis posterior tendon, the deltoid ligament, the spring ligament, and the talonavicular capsule. (The spring ligament is considered a plantar structure.) The fibrosis of the above structures form a mass of indistinguishable scar, which obscures the midtarsal and subtalar joints, and maintain the tuberosity of the navicular and the sustentaculum tali in close proximity to the medial malleolus. These are the shortened fibroelastic components of the talocalcaneonavicular joint that cause the "atresia" of the acetabulum described by Brockman.[5] In the resistant foot, this mass of scar tissue prevents the forward and lateral migration of the navicular and the eversion and lateral movement of the anterior end of the calcaneus, which are necessary to restore normal tarsal relationships and correct the deformity. In the severe deformity, where the navicular and sustentaculum tali almost articulate with the medial malleolus, a thick fibrocartilagenous disc is often interposed between the malleolus and the tarsal bones. This abnormality has also been reported by Kleiger.[10]

Tibialis posterior muscle. This muscle is shortened, and its sheath is usually quite hypertrophied. Just distal to the medial malleolus, the tendon loses its normal cylindrical shape and immediately blends with the common mass of scar tissue

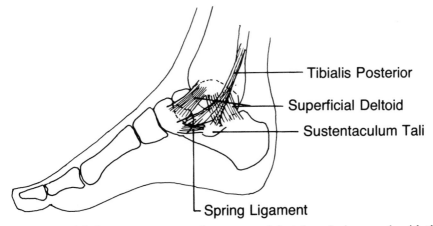

Tibialis Posterior

Superficial Deltoid

Sustentaculum Tali

Spring Ligament

Fig. 4-17. Medial plantar contractures. Contracture of the talonavicular capsule with the above contractures form a medial mass of scar tissue interposed between the malleolus above and the navicular and sustentaculum below.

noted previously. It must be recalled that the tibialis posterior attaches to the spring ligament, the sustentaculum tali, and the navicular. One must also keep in mind that not only is this muscle shortened, but its tendon insertions are also abnormal and contribute to the resistance.

The flexor digitorum longus and flexor hallicus longus. Both of these muscles are shortened. The shortening per se does not contribute to the basic clubfoot deformity, since these muscles insert on the toes; shortened flexor tendons will cause a flexion contracture of the toes without affecting the tarsal relationship. The flexor tendon sheaths cross the midtarsal and subtalar joints, and if sufficiently contracted and thickened, they can add to the resistance. The contracted Henry's knot (the annular ligament for the two flexor tendons) is an important plantar collagen contracture that restricts the mobility of the navicular by virtue of its attachment to the undersurface of the navicular.

The plantar calcaneonavicular ligament (spring ligament). This ligament is always contracted and may even be displaced medially from its normal plantar position under the talar head. It becomes shortened and inelastic because in the equinovarus position the navicular is closer to the sustentaculum tali, and the spring ligament is relaxed. With persistent deformity this fibroelastic structure becomes a contracture that prevents forward and lateral movement of the navicular and also contributes to the atresia of the socket that contains the head of the talus.

Talonavicular capsule. As with the spring ligament, the medial part of the talonavicular capsule becomes a shortened contracture secondary to its lax state in the varus position. In cases where there is slight dorsal subluxation of the navicular, the dorsal part of this capsule may be also contracted.

Subtalar Contractures. *(Talocalcaneal interosseous ligament, bifurcated "Y" ligament)*

Fibrosis and shortening of the talocalcaneal interosseous ligament contracture (Fig. 4-18) increases with age and with the degree of varus. In the younger child,

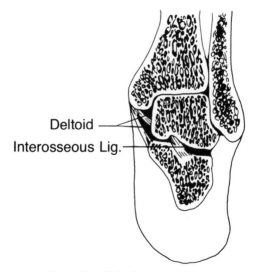

Deltoid
Interosseous Lig.

Fig. 4-18.   Subtalar contractures.

especially under 1 year of age, this structure may be only minimally shortened. In the older child, this ligament may appear as an extremely thickened, dense mass of rigid scar tissue that firmly binds together the calcaneus and the talus. Contractures of the bifurcated (Y) ligament, although less common, can prevent complete correction of the varus adduction components in some severe deformities.

Plantar Contractures (Cavus). *(Abductor hallucis, intrinsic toe flexors, quadratus plantae, plantar aponeurosis)*

As noted previously, a cavus deformity (Fig. 4-19) is present in some of the infants with a severe deformity; it is commonly seen in the older child with an uncorrected clubfoot. The soft-tissue contractures associated with a flexion deformity of the forefoot include: the plantar aponeurosis, abductor hallucis, the intrinsic toe flexors, the quadratus, and the deep plantar ligaments. The plantar aponeurosis is invariably contracted and is palpable as a tight, subcutaneous fibrous band along the medial plantar surface of the foot in the older child. Contracture of the plantar aponeurosis is less prominent in children less than 4 years old.

The abductor hallucis normally arises from the medial plantar surface of the calcaneus. In a severe cavus deformity, it has an accessory abnormal attachment-of-origin from the tendon sheaths of the tibialis posterior, the sheaths of the two flexor tendons, and the navicular tuberosity. The intrinsic toe flexors are shortened as a result of an adaptation to the varus and adduction deformity (shortened medial border of the foot). The first metatarsal is usually plantar flexed. It is common to find a broad accessory insertion of the **anterior tibial tendon** distally on the shaft of the first metatarsal in patients with a cavus component. The insertion may extend down to the midshaft of the first metatarsal.

The calf and extrinsic muscles. The calf is atrophied and diminished in bulk, with shortening of the triceps, posterior tibial, and both long toe flexors. The discrepancy in the size of the calf musculature becomes more obvious as the child grows. The most severe degree of calf atrophy, stork-like legs, are seen in patients with deformities that resemble arthrogryposis, and in children who have had re-

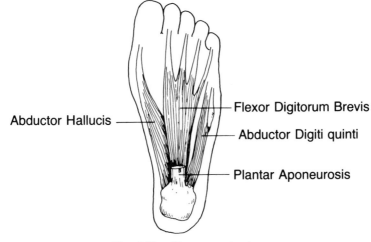

Abductor Hallucis

Flexor Digitorum Brevis

Abductor Digiti quinti

Plantar Aponeurosis

Fig. 4-19.   Plantar contractures.

peated or excessive heel-cord lengthening operations. The peroneals are usually elongated and exhibit varying degrees of weakness. (Clinically this can only be ascertained in older children.) Most studies involving routine microscopic investigations[9,15] have found no abnormalities in the muscles, nerves, and blood vessels.

Abnormal tendon and muscle attachments. Some investigators have reported "no abnormal tendon attachments" in dissections of stillborn and neonatal specimens. In contrast, I have repeatedly observed, at surgery, abnormal accessory attachments of the tibialis posterior, the achilles tendon, and the tibialis anterior. An abnormal origin of the abductor hallucis muscle is common in feet with severe cavus. The postnatal development of these abnormalities represents adaptive changes that result from accessory attachments to displaced bones in the immediate vicinity of these soft tissues. Tendons and muscles have an inherent tendency to attach themselves to adjacent bones; it is significant to note that abnormal tendon attachments also occur in severe planovalgus deformities. In children with a severe flatfoot, it is not unusual to find the tendo achilles inserting more laterally on the valgus heel, whereas in children with clubfoot the Achilles inserts more medially on the inverted heel. This reinforces the hypothesis that abnormal tendon attachments may be secondary to bony deformity. In my experience, abnormal tendon insertions are not unusual in clubfeet and are more prevelant in the severe deformities and in older children.

SUMMARY

The basic anatomic derangement in clubfoot is a congenital subluxation of the talocalcaneonavicular joint in which the navicular and the calcaneus are displaced medially in relation to the talus. An increased medial deviation and deformity of the neck and head of the talus are consistent findings; contracted rigid soft tissues resist the correction of the abnormal tarsal relationship. Some of the osseous and soft tissue abnormalities are acquired. Pathologic anatomy varies from patient to patient case, depending on the severity of the deformity, the age of the patient, and prior treatment. The ankle, subtalar joints, and midtarsal joints are involved in the deformity. The essential morbid anatomy lies in the talocalcaneonavicular complex; the forefoot deformity also contributes in part to the composite deformity.

For purposes of treatment, it is essential to appreciate that the clubfoot deformity is a composite of equinus, varus, and adduction components; at times, cavus is also present. Equinus, varus, and adduction occur simultaneously and not as separate independent components. Plantar flexion is accompanied by supination, and in the clubfoot this is a fixed deformity. Dorsiflexion is a combination of upward movement of the talus in the ankle joint, accompanied by simultaneous eversion in the talocalcaneonavicular complex. In the clubfoot, dorsiflexion is prevented by the unyielding contracted fibroelastic structures that comprise the socket for the head of the talus. These rigid structures prevent both lateral movement of the navicular and dorsiflexion and eversion of the calcaneus. Because of the interrelationship of dorsiflexion and pronation, it is impossible to completely correct one component of the deformity without, at the same time, eliminating the others. The calcaneus per se is fixed in equinus, varus, and adduction.

REFERENCES

1. Adams, W.: Clubfoot: Its Causes, Pathology and Treatment. J. and A. Churchill, London, 1866.
2. Attenborough, C. G.: Congenital talipes equinovarus. Journal of Bone and Joint Surgery, *48B*:31-39, 1966.
3. Bissell, J. B.: Anatomy of congenital talipes equinovarus. Archives of Pediatrics, 406-418, 1888.
4. Bost, F. C., Schottstadt, E. R., and Larsen, L. J.: Plantar dissection—an operation to release the soft tissues in recurrent talipes equinovarus. Journal of Bone and Joint Surgery, *42A*:151, 1960.
5. Brockman, E. P.: Congenital Clubfoot. John Wright and Sons, Bristol, 1930.
6. Elmsie, R. C.: Principles in treatment of congenital talipes equinovarus. Journal of Orthopedic Surgery, *2*:669, 1920.
7. Evans, D.: Relapsed clubfoot. Journal of Bone and Joint Diseases, *43B*: 1961.
8. Goldner, J. L.: Congenital Talipes Equinovarus—Fifteen-Year Surgical Treatment. Current Practice in Orthopedic Surgery. Vol. 4. C. V. Mosby, St. Louis, 1962.
9. Irani, R. N., and Sherman, M. S.: The pathological anatomy of clubfoot. Journal of Bone and Joint Surgery, *45A,* Jan. 1963.
10. Kleiger, B.: The Significance of tibio talar navicular complex in congenital clubfoot. Bulletin of the Hospital for Joint Diseases, *23*:158-69, 1962.
11. Little, W. J.: A Treatise on the Nature of Clubfoot and Analogous Distortions. London, 1839.
12. McCauley, J. C.: Surgical treatment of clubfeet. Surgical Clinics of North America, *3*:561, 1951.
13. Scarpa, A.: A Memoir on the Congenital Clubfeet of Children. (Translated by J. W. Wishart). Constable, Edinburgh, 1818.
14. Schlicht, D.: The pathological anatomy of talipes equinovarus. Australian-New Zealand Journal of Surgery, *33*:2-11, 1963.
15. Stewart, S. F.: Clubfoot: Its incidence, cause and treatment. Journal of Bone and Joint Surgery, *33A,* No. 3, 1951.
16. Swann, M., Lloyd-Roberts, G. C., and Caterall, A.: The anatomy of uncorrected clubfoot. A study of rotation deformity. *51B,* May 1969.
17. Turco, V. J.: Resistant congenital clubfoot. American Academy of Orthopaedic Surgeons Instructional Course Lectures, vol. 24. The C. V. Mosby Co., St. Louis, 1975.
18. Wiley, A. M.: An anatomical and experimental study of muscle growth in clubfeet. Journal of Bone and Joint Surgery. 41B, Nov. 1958.

5 | Radiology

OSSIFICATION

In the normal foot at birth, the centers of ossification for the talus, calcaneus, and metatarsals are visible, and that for the cuboid may also be present. Ossification of the cuneiforms appears later; the lateral ossifies first, the middle second, and the medial cuneiform third. The navicular is the last tarsal bone to ossify.

In the clubfoot, the appearance of the centers of ossification for the tarsal bones is usually delayed. The ossified nucleus of the navicular appears much later in the clubfoot than in the normal foot; it may not appear until the child is 4 or, in some cases, even 5 or 6 years old. I believe that ossification of the navicular in the clubfoot is significantly retarded because the abnormal tarsal relationship at the talonavicular joint fails to provide the normal physiologic stimulus on the navicular. In older children (4 to 6 years old), I have observed that ossification of the navicular frequently appears shortly after the normal tarsal relationship has been restored. I also have observed that, in some of the older children, the ossific nucleus of the navicular is quite small preoperatively; it usually enlarges shortly after the talonavicular subluxation is surgically reduced. The onset of ossification and the increase in size of the navicular ossification nucleus shortly after the deformity is corrected suggest a response to normal mechanics and physiologic stress (Wolff's law); this occurrence can also be utilized as additional evidence that the normal tarsal relationship has been restored.

RADIOGRAPHS

Neonatal Period. In the clubfoot at birth, only the ossification centers of the talus, the calcaneus, and the metatarsals are usually present. The two tarsal bones appear as small rounded ossicles, and for this reason radiographs taken in the neonatal period add very little to the information gained from the clinical

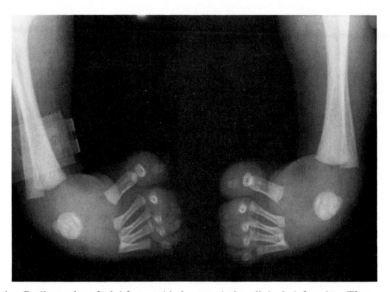

Fig. 5-1. Radiographs of clubfeet at birth record the clinical deformity. They are not, however, informative regarding the shape and orientation of the tarsal bones. The only ossification centers present are those of the talus, calcaneus, and metatarsals; rarely, the nucleus of the cuboid is present. The small, rounded ossific nuclei of the talus and calcaneus represent a very small portion of the tarsal bones and are not necessarily the centers of these anlagen.

examination. At this age, radiographic examination is not informative or revealing, because the presence of two small, round ossific nuclei on the x-ray film does not help to evaluate the shape and orientation of the tarsal anlagen. In addition, it is virtually impossible to hold the neonate's foot in the proper position for a meaningful examination; the holder's hand would obscure the bones.

Radiographs taken at birth are useful in detecting osseous anomalies such as teratogenic defects and provide a good record of the deformity. Most of the tarsus is unossified at birth and therefore invisible on the x-ray film. Only the small ossification center, which, in the neonate, does not reveal the abnormal shape or relationship of the cartilaginous anlagen, can be seen on the radiograph. The medial inclination of the neck of the talus, the deformity of the head of the talus, and the talonavicular relationship are not visible until these parts of the cartilaginous anlagen are sufficiently ossified.

In summary, radiographic examination of the clubfoot in the neonatal period reveals only small ossification masses, which are not a manifestation of the shape or orientation of the bones. One should also bear in mind that the initial, visible ossification center does not necessarily represent the anatomic center of each tarsal bone and that, the younger the child, the less informative the study is (Fig. 5-1).

Radiographs During Infancy. I do not mean to imply, from the preceding remarks, that radiographic examinations are valueless in the treatment of clubfoot. On the contrary, radiographs taken during infancy are very informative and valuable in assessing the correction. At 2 to 3 months of age, the anlagen for the talus and that for the calcaneus are still predominantly cartilagenous. However,

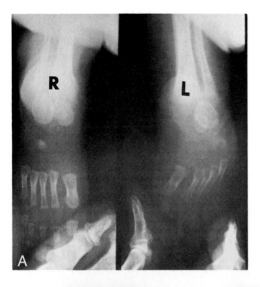

Fig. 5-2. A 10-week-old infant with a left clubfoot. *(A),* At 2 to 3 months of age, the long axes of the ossified nuclei of the talus and calcaneus provide useful information regarding the tarsal relationship. One should note that there is less divergence of the hindfoot and that the bones (especially the talus) are smaller in the left clubfoot.

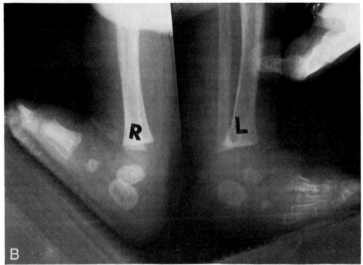

Fig. 5-2. *(B),* Comparison dorsiflexion lateral radiographs demonstrate the abnormal relationships between the talus and calcaneus and between the tibia and calcaneus in the clubfoot.

sufficient ossification is present at this time so that radiographs provide useful information. During infancy, the ossification centers are a poor guide to the shape of the bones, but ossification is sufficient to ascertain the long axes of the talus and the calcaneus. These long axes usually provide a fairly accurate impression of the relationship between the calcaneus and the talus and their relationship to the ankle joint [Fig. 5-2 *(A, B)*]. This is especially true for the calcaneus, the mature form of which is outlined at an early age, long before the talus. The mature form of the talus cannot be assessed accurately by radiographic examination until

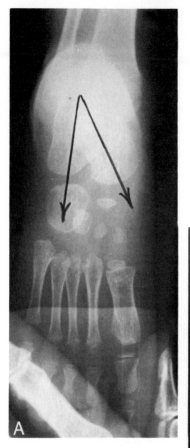

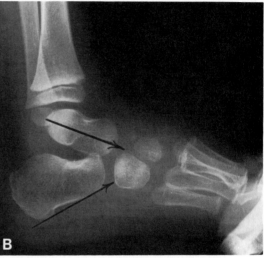

Fig. 5-3. Normal foot. *(A)*, In the anteroposterior view the long axes of the talus and calcaneus form a divergent angle of about 30°. There is considerable variation within the normal range. Numerical measurement of the talocalcaneal angle can be distorted by the position of the foot on the x-ray cassette and by cephalad angulation of the x-ray tube. The navicular is anterior to the head of the talus. *(B)*, Lateral view. The long axis of the talus points downward and medially. The axis of the calcaneus is directed upward in relation to the tibia, slightly lateral in the sagittal plane. The numerical measurement of the talocalcaneal angle is affected by the degree of dorsiflexion and plantar flexion.

the child begins to attain skeletal maturity. In my experience, radiographs taken during infancy provided a helpful, valuable method for evaluating responses to treatment. Both the information obtained and the value of radiologic evaluation improve as ossification of the tarsal anlagen increases with growth.

Normal Talocalcaneal Relationship. In the anteroposterior view of the normal foot, the long axes of the talus and the calcaneus form a divergent angle [Fig. 5-3 *(A)*], which is increased in the planovalgus foot and decreased with equinovarus deformity; this relationship changes during normal growth and development of the foot. The talocalcaneal angle of divergence is widest in the newborn and gradually lessens up to the age of 6 or 7 years.[4] This may be one of the reasons why pes planus is common in infancy and gradually disappears with growth as the talocalcaneal angle diminishes and the child develops an arch. The talocalcaneal angle remains more divergent in children who have a persistent pes planus.

In the lateral projection, the long axis of the talus is downward while that of the calcaneus is upward [Fig. 5-3 *(B)*]. In the normal foot, dorsiflexion is greatest at birth and, like the physiologic pes planus, gradually decreases with growth. The stress dorsiflexion lateral radiograph of a normal foot will show decreasing dorsiflexion up to age 6 or 7 years. Similarly, in the corrected clubfoot, the degree of dorsiflexion will gradually diminish with maturity.

Slight, gradual loss of dorsiflexion following correction of the clubfoot is to be expected and is considered a normal occurrence, similar to the progressively diminishing dorsiflexion associated with growth and development of the normal foot. The talocalcaneal angle, as measured in the lateral projection, varies with the degree of dorsiflexion and plantarflexion; the angle increases with dorsiflexion and lessens in plantar flexion. In plantar flexion, the talus and calcaneus assume a more parallel relationship to each other. In addition to the variations associated with the normal growth, development, and position of the foot, the limits of normal also vary widely. Some normal children have wider angles of divergence in the anteroposterior view or increased plantar flexion of the talus, which is commonly seen in children with pes planus.

Some authors have made radiologic assessments by measuring the talocalcaneal angles in the anteroposterior and the lateral projections.[1,2,4,5] I have not used this method for assessing correction because there is a wide range of variation within the limits of normal; normal values will vary depending on the child's age; drawing lines through the middle of a small ossified mass is inaccurate, especially since the mass is not necessarily the center of the bone; furthermore, the degree of dorsiflexion or plantar flexion and the adduction of the leg significantly affect the measurements.*

Arthrography. To date, the use of arthrography in clubfoot has not been successful. It is possible to inject contrast media into the ankle joint and get an outline of the intraarticular portion of the body of the talus. However, arthrography of the ankle joint merely confirms what is already known—i.e., that the posterior part of the trochlea is in the mortise; that the apparent extrusion of the talus anteriorly, out of the mortise, is due to plantar flexion; and that ossification of the talus starts eccentrically in the anterior part. Attempts to outline the head and the neck of the talus and the position of the navicular by injecting dye into the talonavicular joint have proved technically very difficult and unsatisfactory. Injection of the subtalar joint has also been nonproductive. The abnormal tarsal relationship, marked loss of joint space in the midtarsal and subtalar joints, plus the atresia and fibrosis of the talocalcaneonavicular socket make it virtually impossible to obtain a satisfactory arthrographic study to warrant the risk of iatrogenic damage. On the basis of the pathologic anatomy noted at surgery, one can readily understand why arthrography to date has failed to add to the knowledge gained by radiographic and clinical examinations.

Radiologic Evaluation. It is my opinion that radiologic assessment of the correction is more reliable and gives a more accurate objective record than does clinical evaluation. Properly taken radiographs avoid a false clinical impression of an apparent correction. Clinically, the heel varus may appear to be corrected because manipulations have displaced the heel pad laterally, whereas radiographs will demonstrate an abnormal tarsal relationship between the calcaneus and talus, thus confirming the fact that one is dealing with a spurious correction.

---

* McKinnon and coworkers[3] have shown that numerical measurement of talocalcaneal angles can be significantly distorted by the position of the foot and the angle of the x-ray beam. Since it is very difficult to precisely position a child's deformed foot, measurements of talocalcaneal angles can be easily distorted. Distortion of numerical measurement of the talocalcaneal angle is potentially greater in the anteroposterior radiograph because the x-ray tube must be angled cephalad in order to visualize the hindfoot; also, slight adduction of the leg will produce an apparent divergence of the hindfoot,

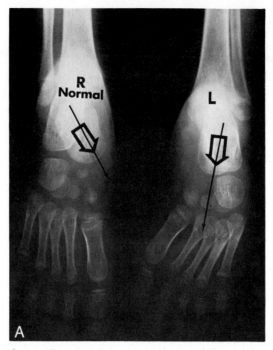

Fig. 5-4. Left clubfoot with comparison views of normal foot. *(A),* In the left clubfoot the talus and calcaneus are superimposed on each other, and there is less divergence than in the normal. Continuation of a line drawn through the long axis of the talus falls over the second metatarsal rather than medial to the first metatarsal as in the normal foot. This lateral deviation increases with the degree of heel varus and forefoot adduction. Navicular ossification is present in the normal foot and delayed in the clubfoot. One should note that the calcaneocuboid joints are symmetrical, and there is no apparent medial displacement of the cuboid in the clubfoot. Note how adduction of the forefoot at the Lisfranc level contributes to the composite adduction varus deformity.

In the unilateral deformity, the clubfoot should be compared to the normal foot. The ossification centers in the very small infant do not show the shape of the bones; ossification must be sufficient to provide a rudimentary outline of the shape of the tarsal bones. As I stated earlier, the degree of correction cannot be assessed accurately by measuring the talocalcaneal angles because the limits of normal vary widely, values differ with age, degrees of dorsi and plantar flexion differ, and, finally, it is inaccurate to assume that a line drawn through the ossification represents the center and configuration of the bone. As in clinical findings, radiographic findings will vary according to the age of the patient, the severity of the deformity, and prior treatment. These variations must constantly be kept in mind as the radiographs are correlated with these factors. The radiographic examination is based on the normal anatomy and the mechanics of dorsiflexion and plantar flexion of the foot.

---

or increase the talocalcaneal angle. Angle distortion is more magnified in the uncorrected foot than in the normal. For the previously stated reasons, in my opinion radiologic analysis of correction based on a numerical addition of the biocalcaneal angles of the lateral and anteroposterior radiographs is a potential source of misleading information.

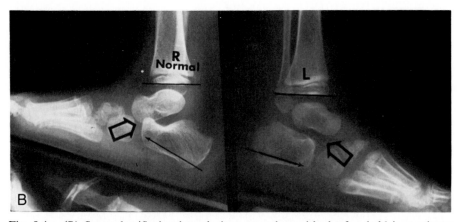

Fig. 5-4. *(B),* Stress dorsiflexion lateral views are taken with the feet held in maximum dorsiflexion by a board under the plantar surface of the feet. In the normal foot, as the calcaneus dorsiflexes, the tibiocalcaneal angle is increased and there is overlapping of the distal ends of the calcaneus and talus. One should also note the rounded anterior body of the talus and constriction of the talar neck. In the uncorrected left clubfoot there is no dorsiflexion of the calcaneus in relation to the tibia. The talus and calcaneus are parallel, and there is no overlap of the anterior ends of the calcaneus and talus; the sinus tarsi remain open. Some of the limited dorsiflexion is attributable to impingement of the overgrown anterior portion of the body and neck of the talus on the anterior lip of the tibia. The usual posterior displacement of the fibula is exaggerated by stabilizing the convex lateral border of the forefoot on the cassette by rotating the foot laterally.

The anteroposterior view [Fig. 5-4 (A)]. As stated previously, in the normal foot there is a divergence of the long axes of the talus and calcaneus. Therefore the long axis of the talus, when drawn through the middle of the ossified nucleus, is directed medial to the first metatarsal. In the clubfoot, the angle of divergence is diminished; because the calcaneus is inverted, and because its anterior end is adducted under the talus, the talus and calcaneus appear to be superimposed on each other. The continuation of the long axis of the talus falls lateral to the first metatarsal as a result of the inversion, adduction deformity of the heel, and the forefoot adduction. In a severe deformity, the calcaneus and talus may be completely superimposed on each other. Except for the assessment of hindfoot divergence, the anteroposterior view is of limited value because the medially displaced navicular cannot be detected until ossification occurs. (The navicular is the last bone to ossify and ossification is even more delayed in the clubfoot as compared with the normal foot). After the navicular ossifies, its medial displacement is obvious in the uncorrected foot of the older child.

The lateral view [Fig. 5-4(B)]. The foot is held in a position of maximum dorsiflexion for this view. The rational of this technique is based on the normal mechanics of dorsiflexion, which results from movement in the ankle and in the talocalcaneonavicular joints. In dorsiflexion, the posterior tuberosity of the calcaneus moves downward as the anterior end everts and moves upward. At the same time, the navicular must be free to move laterally in unison with the anterior end of the calcaneus around the head of the talus. In the uncorrected clubfoot, the calcaneus is locked in varus under the talus, and the navicular is bound medially by soft tissue contractures. Therefore in the lateral dorsiflexion projection, one sees persistent equinus with the inability of the calcaneus to dorsiflex. The three signs of persistent equinovarus deformity are: (1) no dorsiflexion of the heel in relation to the ankle joint; (2) parallelism of the talus and calcaneus; and (3) no overlap of the anterior ends of the calcaneus and talus (the sinus tarsi is still open). In the radiograph, the posterior displacement of the fibula is exaggerated. This occurs because the technician stabilizes a convex lateral border of the foot by keeping the forefoot flat on the cassette, thereby further increasing the external rotation of the ankle mortise.

It can be shown that the calcaneus is locked under the talus by comparing the relationship of the talus and the calcaneus in lateral radiographs taken with the foot held in full dorsiflexion and plantar flexion. These radiographs will show that the talocalcaneal angle remains the same in a clubfoot but increases when the normal foot is dorsiflexed [Fig. 5-5*(A,B,C)*].

Technique.   Both feet must be held in identical positions for an accurate meaningful radiographic assessment.

For the anteroposterior view, the knee, leg, and foot must be in the vertical position. The technician may find it easier to stabilize the inverted deformed foot by adducting the leg. However, this position will produce a false, apparent divergence of the hindfoot [Fig. 5-6*(A,B)*]. In the infant, it is very difficult to stabilize and maintain proper positioning of the feet. Therefore, symmetric positioning is best attained by having the mother hold the infant's knees together, keeping the infant's legs flexed and his feet resting on the cassette in 20° to 30° of plantar flexion. The x-ray tube is directed 20° cephalad in order to visualize the talus and the calcaneus [Fig. 5–6*(C,D)*].

For the older child, radiographs are taken with the child sitting on a small stool, with his knees bent and his ankles in slight plantar flexion so that the hindfoot can be properly visualized. With an extremely severe equinus deformity, the anteroposterior projection may produce an apparent divergence of the hindfoot, because in equinus the medial inclination of the long axis of the talus is exaggerated.

(continued on page 70)

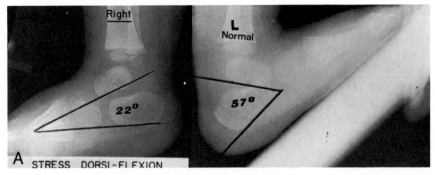

Fig. 5-5.   Right clubfoot with comparison views of the patient's normal foot. *(A)*, Dorsiflexion lateral views of right clubfoot and left normal foot show that the talocalcaneal and the tibiocalcaneal angles are diminished in the right clubfoot.

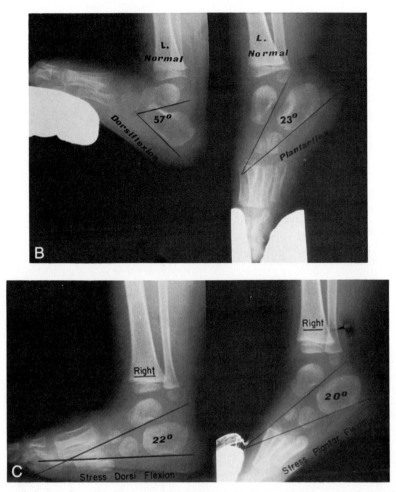

Fig. 5-5 *(continued)*. *(B)*, The normal left foot held in dorsiflexion and plantar flexion demonstrates a significant change of the talocalcaneal angle with vertical movement. When the calcaneus is dorsiflexed, its posterior end moves downward as the anterior end everts and moves upward; hence the talocalcaneal angle in dorsiflexion is increased. In the plantar-flexed position, the talocalcaneal angle is diminished as the calcaneus assumes a more parallel relationship with the talus and inverts under the talus. Note that in plantar flexion the talocalcaneal angle of the normal foot is quite similar to that of the clubfoot [Fig. 5-5 *(C)*]. *(C)*, The right clubfoot held in maximum dorsiflexion and plantar flexion. Note that the parallel relationship between the talus and calcaneus remains the same. The talocalcaneal angle does not change because the calcaneus is locked in varus under the talus by soft tissue contractures, which prevent eversion of the calcaneus and downward movement of its posterior tuberosity. The limited vertical motion takes place solely in the ankle. Full dorsiflexion of the ankle is limited by the incongruity between the anterior talus and the anterior lip of the tibia. Note that the talocalcaneal angle of the clubfoot is similar to that of the normal foot in plantar flexion [Fig. 5.5 *(B)*].

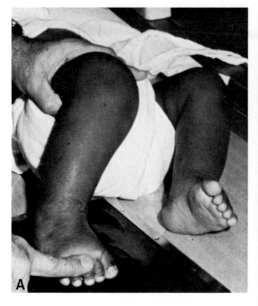

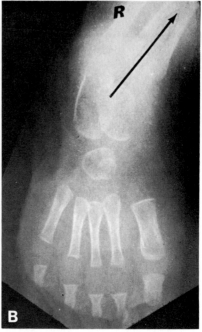

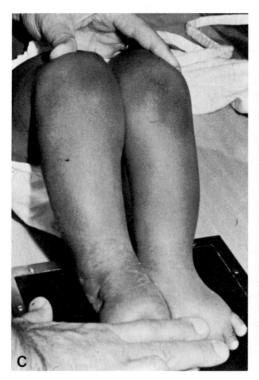

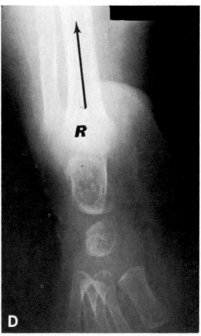

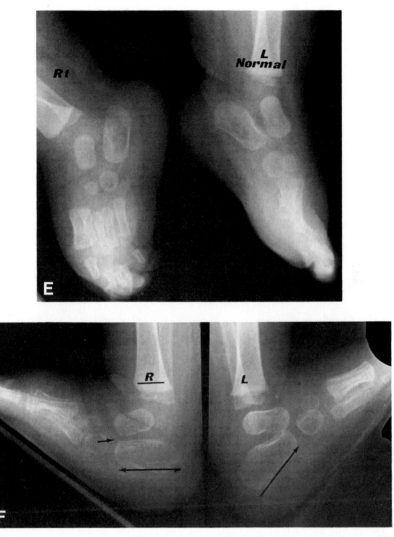

Fig. 5-6. Radiographic technique—right clubfoot. *(A),* The leg is placed in an adducted position. An anteroposterior view *(B),* taken with the leg adducted, produced a distorted relationship with apparent divergence of the calcaneus and talus. Such a divergence of the hindfoot can also be produced by increasing the cephalad angulation of the x-ray tube. *(C),* The knee, leg, and foot are placed in a vertical position. With proper positioning of the same foot, the radiograph *(D),* reveals that the talus and calcaneus are superimposed. *(E),* Lateral views taken with both feet in plantar flexion produced a radiograph in which the clubfoot appears similar to the normal foot. *(F),* Lateral views taken with the feet forced into maximum dorsiflexion by a board on the plantar surface clearly show the difference between the uncorrected and normal foot. The dorsiflexion lateral view of the right clubfoot reveals the absence of calcaneal dorsiflexion in relation to the tibia. Assessment of the tibiocalcaneal angle is the most reliable method for evaluating correction. The x-ray tube is directed at a right angle to the foot.

Another possible explanation is that the ossific nucleus of the talus may be more medially eccentric, thereby contributing to the illusion of apparent divergence of the hindfoot.

A lateral view, taken with the foot in the equinus position, is of no value because the clubfoot will be indistinguishable from the normal one [Fig. 5–6(E)]. The lateral view is taken with the foot held in a maximum dorsiflexed position by a piece of wood 2 cm thick. This study is the most accurate and reliable for evaluating the correction [Fig. 5–6(F)].

The anteroposterior view is of a limited value because the navicular is not ossified. A critical review of the lateral radiograph in cases of recurrent deformity usually reveals that heel dorsiflexion was never attained. It is not unusual to see cases in which the anteroposterior radiograph shows an apparent correction, as evidenced by hindfoot divergence, but the dorsiflexion lateral view shows no dorsiflexion of the calcaneus. In these instances, the findings at surgery proved the accuracy of the dorsiflexion lateral x-ray view (Fig. 5-7). However, findings will vary depending on the patient's age and the severity of the deformity (Fig. 5-8).

Rocker-Bottom Deformity. A rocker-bottom is an iatrogenic deformity that results from persistent vigorous attempts to dorsiflex and evert the foot in the presence of unyielding soft-tissue contractures. I have not seen this deformity in an untreated clubfoot. Rigid contractures prevent motion at the midtarsal and subtalar joints, and in addition it is difficult to apply an effective corrective force on the heel and the navicular. In contrast, contractures at the tarsometatarsal joints are more pliable. Thus, the force applied to the forefoot is more effective, since this part of the foot can be grasped firmly and provides a long lever arm. With repeated manipulations, therefore, a breech occurs at the tarsometatarsal joints, resulting in dorsiflexion and abduction of the forefoot and a convex plantar surface (Fig. 5-9). Hypermobility occurs at the Lisfranc joints. Repeatedly, in surgery of rocker-bottom feet I have noted extremely dense, medial-plantar contractures without hypermobility of the midtarsal joint, which would be expected if the breach occurred at the talonavicular level. Also, the navicular and the sustentaculum tali frequently are completely displaced medially and held by a dense mass of unyielding fibrous tissue. Occasionally, the navicular may be slightly dorsal to the head of the talus, but it is always displaced medially. (This displacement has also been noted in nonrocker-bottom clubfeet.) Just as frequently, the posterior body of the talus appeared wafer thin at surgery because of the marked plantar flexion of the talus.

Clinically, the foot may appear corrected because the forefoot abduction obscures the dorsolateral prominence of the uncovered head of the talus. However, a spurious correction of the equinus occurs because the forefoot is forced into dorsiflexion; the heel pad is displaced laterally causing an apparent correction of heel varus. It has been observed that in the child with a unilateral clubfoot with a rocker-bottom, the normal foot is severely flat.

The anteroposterior radiograph invariably shows apparent divergence of the hindfoot. Close scrutiny of the film reveals that the forefoot is abducted and the continuation of a line drawn along the lateral border of the calcaneus and cuboid crosses the midmetatarsal area [Fig. 5-9(D)]. The lateral radiograph shows no

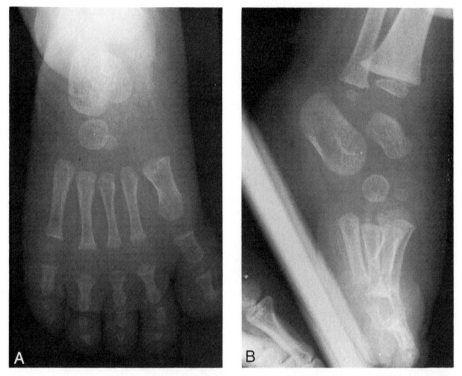

Fig. 5-7.   Clubfoot at age 15 months. *(A)*, This case example illustrates a clubfoot in which the anteroposterior view may show an apparent divergence of the hindfoot. At surgery, however, the calcaneus was found inverted under the talus. Since the ossific nucleus of the navicular is absent, it was impossible to assess the medial displacement of this bone, which was noted at surgery. *(B)*, The dorsiflexion lateral view reveals a fixed equinus deformity with inability of the calcaneus to dorsiflex in spite of the apparent correction in the anteroposterior view. This lateral view provides a more accurate method of assessing the correction. It is difficult to distort the dorsiflexion lateral view because the x-ray beam is directed perpendicular to the talus and calcaneus which lie in the same plane on the x-ray cassette. Distortion of the hindfoot divergence is potentially greater in the anteroposterior view for the following reasons: the talus and calcaneus are not in the same plane; the talus is closer to the x-ray tube and farther away from the cassette than the calcaneus; and in equinus the medial angulation of the talus is increased. Therefore, the anteroposterior view taken with cephalad angulation of the x-ray tube can distort the medial deviation of the talus and produce an apparent normal divergence of the hindfoot, as evidenced in this case. Note that in the lateral view the talus appears subluxed out of the mortise and its anterior end is distal to the calcaneus, whereas in the anteroposterior view the talus appears to be located proximal to the calcaneus. While looking at the lateral view, one should visualize the x-ray beam directed cephalad for the anteroposterior view. This angle distortion produces the apparent hindfoot divergence shown in Fig. 5.7 *(A)*. This distortion in the anteroposterior view is magnified in cases with a greater degree of plantar flexion of the talus, by holding the foot in more equinus or by increasing the cephalad angulation of the x-ray tube.

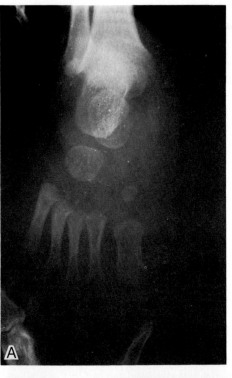

Fig. 5-8.   Uncorrected right clubfoot at 2 years *(A,B)* and 6 years of age *(C,D, facing page) (A)*, At 2 years of age, the anteroposterior view shows apparent correction, and the calcaneus and talus appear to be diverted. Absence of navicular ossification makes it impossible to assess its position in relation to talus. *(B)*, At 2 years of age the lateral view shows there is no dorsiflexion of the calcaneus with parallelism of the hindfoot. The significance of the absence of calcaneal dorsiflexion was not appreciated at this time.

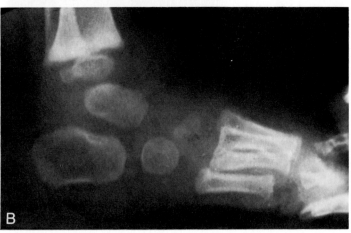

dorsiflexion of the calcaneus, and the talus is plantar flexed much more than usual. Occasionally this deformity, in the toddler, is mistaken for a congenital plantar-flexed talus, which is differentiated in a lateral radiograph taken with the foot held in plantar flexion.

Cavus Deformity (Fig. 5-10). A cavus deformity is readily recognized in the lateral projection by plantar flexion of the first metatarsal. This is usually more obvious and evident in the older child, although it can also be seen, to a

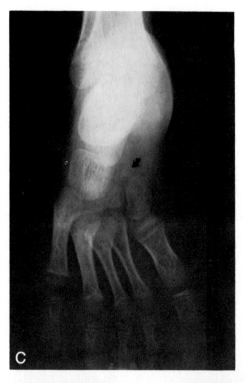

Fig. 5-8 *(continued).* *(C),* At 6 years of age, increased ossification of the anlagen of the talus and calcaneus shows obvious superimposition of the hindfoot. Note that the ossific nucleus of the navicular is very small and displaced medially in relation to the talar head. *(D),* At 6 years of age the lateral view shows a severe cavus with a plantar flexed first metatarsal and adaptive changes of the talus. This was called a relapsed deformity. Review of the lateral radiographs at 2 years of age revealed that in fact the deformity had not been corrected. This case illustrates the reliability of the dorsiflexion lateral view in assessing correction. Again one should note that ossification of the navicular is markedly delayed in an uncorrected foot.

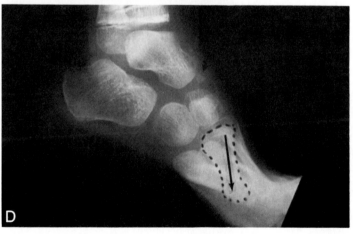

lesser degree, in infancy. The cavus deformity of the clubfoot is distinguished from the idiopathic or neuromuscular cavus by the position of the calcaneus. In the clubfoot, the calcaneus is plantar flexed, whereas in the idiopathic deformity the calcaneus is dorsiflexed.

Flat-Top Talus (Fig. 5-11). The so-called flat-top talus is, in part, an apparent deformity because the body of the talus is visualized in the oblique view. This apparent "flat top" can also be seen in the oblique projection of a normal foot.

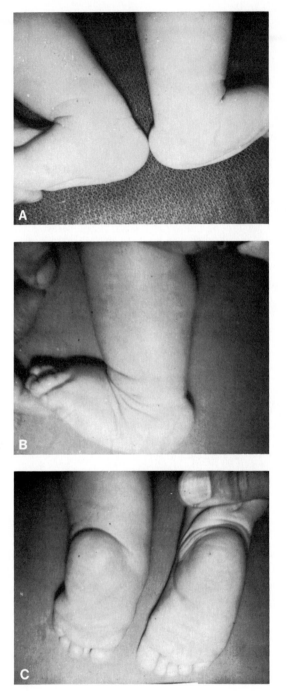

Fig. 5-9. Left rocker-bottom deformity in a 9 month old. *(A),* Medial view. Upward pressure on both feet produces a hyperdorsiflexion of the forefoot with a convex prominence on the plantar surface noted in the left foot similar to a rocking chair—hence the name rocker-bottom. *(B),* Lateral view. The forefoot is easily displaced upward and laterally with very little force. The breach occurs at the hypermobile tarsometatarsal level. Usually the forefoot is rather puffy, swollen, and the skin redundant, as evidenced in this case. *(C),* Plantar view. The heel pad in the left clubfoot has been displaced laterally by manipulations, producing an apparent correction of the heel varus. However, at surgery the calcaneus was found locked in varus under the talus. Note the forefoot abduction of the left foot as compared with the normal right.

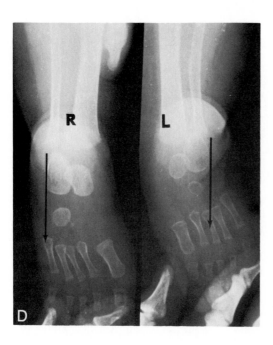

Fig. 5.9 *(continued).* *(D)*, Antero-posterior view shows apparent divergence of the hindfoot. At surgery the navicular was displaced medially. The forefoot is abducted at the tarso-metatarsal joints. One should note that on the left side the continuation of a line drawn along the lateral border of the calcaneus and cuboid falls over the third metatarsal instead of the fifth as in the normal foot. These radiographic abnormalities are the result of manipulations producing hypermobile Lisfranc articulations with an abduction of the forefoot.

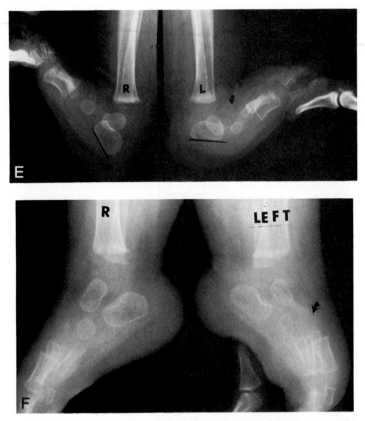

Fig. 5.9 *(continued).* *(E),* The rocker-bottom deformity is easily demonstrated by pushing the forefoot upward. There is no dorsiflexion of the heel in spite of the apparent correction demonstrated in the anteroposterior view. Note the marked plantarflexion of the talus; this is the reason the anteroposterior view in Fig. 5.9*(D)* shows divergence of the hindfoot with an apparent correction of the deformity. The dorsal concavity resembles that seen in a congenital plantar-flexed talus. *(F),* Lateral view in plantar flexion. A rocker-bottom deformity is readily distinguished from a plantar-flexed talus by a lateral view taken with the foot held in forced equinus. Unlike the congenital plantar-flexed talus, in the rocker-bottom the dorsal concavity readily disappears because the dorsolateral deformity at the tarsometatarsal level is quite supple. In a plantar-flexed talus the dorsal concavity does not change in dorsi-flexion and plantar flexion, because the dorsal concavity is caused by unyielding soft tissue contractures over the dorsum of the foot.

The oblique, rather than a true lateral view, is taken because the technician stabilizes the convex lateral border of the foot by forcing the forefoot onto the x-ray cassette, thereby producing an oblique view in which the posterior displacement of the fibula is increased. Another reason for the distortion is the increased external rotation of the ankle mortise, which is even more exaggerated in the older child. When a true lateral view is made by internally rotating the foot, the posterior trochlea of the body of the talus appears dome-shaped. The anterior portion of the talus is deformed by overgrowth of its anterior body and its failure to develop

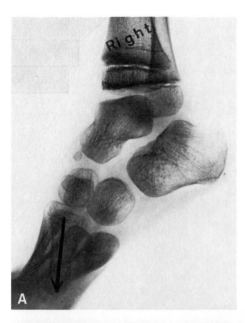

Fig. 5-10. Cavus deformity. *(A)*, Clubfoot cavus. In this deformity, the os calcis is in equinus, the first metatarsal is plantar flexed, the talus is deformed, and the forefoot is plantar flexed. *(B)*, Idiopathic or neuromuscular cavus. In this deformity, the os calcis is dorsiflexed, the shape of the talus is normal, the longitudinal arch is quite high, the metatarsals are in the same alignment, and the toes are usually clawed.

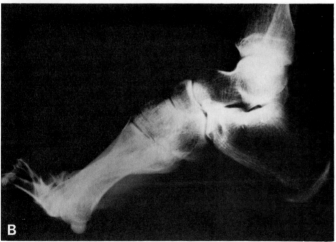

a constriction or neck. The overgrowth in the shape of the talus develops because the anterior portion of the trochlea was never in the mortise and therefore never responded to physiologic stress. The deformity of the anterior part of the talus contributes to the equinus component by impingeing on the anterior lip of the tibia. For this reason, dorsiflexion immediately after posteromedial release may be limited until this part of the talus has an opportunity to remold after correction; this is a reversible abnormality (Fig. 5-12). In the younger child the overgrowth may be a factor in limiting dorsiflexion; however it is not recognized on the x-ray

(continued on page 82)

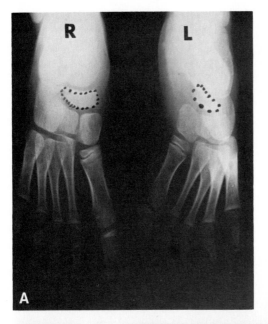

Fig. 5-11. The flat-top talus of an 8 year old with an uncorrected left clubfoot. *(A)*, Anteroposterior view. Left foot shows typical deformity with superimposition of the hindfoot and medially displaced navicular. *(B)*, An oblique view of a clubfoot is taken when the convex lateral border of the foot is stablized by placing the forefoot on the x-ray cassette. This position increases the external rotation of the ankle thereby producing an oblique projection with an apparent flattening of the trochlea of the talus and an apparent deformity of the calcaneus which appears foreshortened with this oblique projection. The posterior displacement of the fibula is also exaggerated by this view.

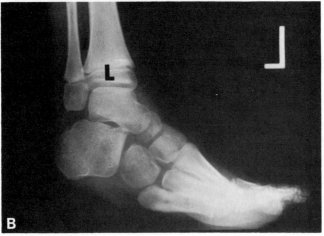

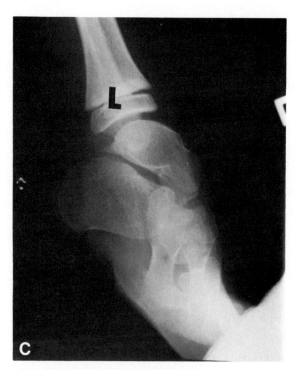

Fig. 5-11 *(continued).   (C)*, Lateral view. A true lateral view is made by internally rotating the foot. The fibula is now in the midline of the tibia. Note that the posterior portion of the trochlea of the talus is in fact rounded and has a normal contour, and the shape of the calcaneus appears normal. A true lateral view demonstrates that plantar flexion of the forefoot contributes to the composite equinus deformity.

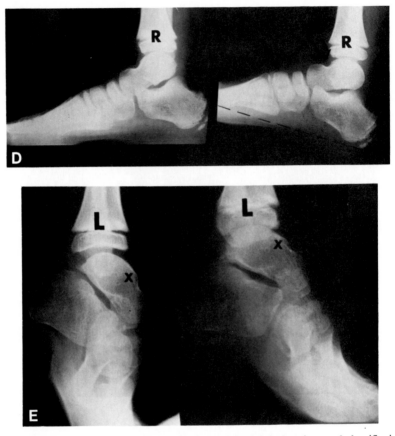

Fig. 5-11 *(continued).* *(D),* Normal right foot with weight-bearing and dorsiflexion. In the neutral weight-bearing position, the normal right foot shows a normally shaped talus. In dorsiflexion, the constricted neck allows all of the round anterior part of the talus to enter the mortise. *(E),* Left clubfoot. In plantar flexion and in dorsiflexion, the posterior portion of the trochlea readily enters the mortise. Since this portion has essentially a normal round configuration, downward movement is unobstructed. The *X* marks the area of the overgrown anterior portion of the trochlea and absent constriction in the talar neck. Some of the limitations of dorsiflexion are caused by the inability of all the trochlea to enter the mortise because this overdeveloped portion of the talus impinges on the anterior lip of the tibia.

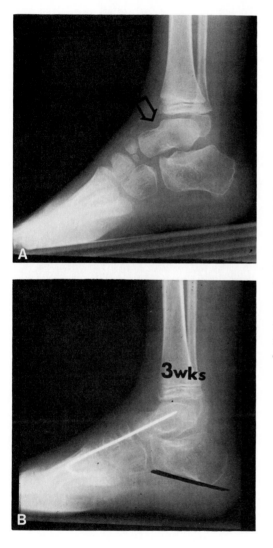

Fig. 5-12. Seven-year old with clubfoot. *(A),* Preoperative radiograph shows typical deformity in the body and neck of the talus. In the older child where more of the anlage is ossified and there is more time to develop adaptive changes, the abnormal shape of the talus is obvious in the radiographs. *(B),* Three weeks after surgical correction dorsiflexion is improved as a little more of the talus can enter the mortise.

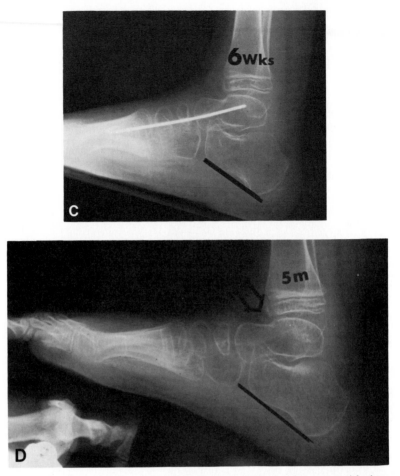

Fig. 5-12 *(continued).*   *(C),* Six weeks after surgery dorsiflexion increases with the gradual remodeling of the talus. *(D),* Five months after surgery the talus demonstrates its capacity to remold to physiological stress before skeletal maturity. With the remodeling of the anterior trochlea and the neck of the talus, full dorsiflexion is now possible because all the talus can enter the mortise. Note that as dorsiflexion increased, the tibiocalcaneal angle also increased.

because this area is still cartilagenous. The deformity becomes evident as ossification increases, and overgrowth of the anterior part of the body and neck of the talus progresses with skeletal development.

SUMMARY

At birth, clinical examination is more informative than radiologic assessment. In infancy, after the tarsal bones have become sufficiently ossified, radiologic evaluation is more reliable and accurate than clinical appraisal. The stress dorsiflexion lateral view, which is based on the normal mechanics of dorsiflexion, is more informative than the anteroposterior projection. Meaningful radiographs demand that the feet be positioned properly for the examination. The rocker-bottom deformity is iatrogenic, occurring at the tarsometatarsal joints following excessive force in the presence of unyielding, rigid soft-tissue contractures that prevent reduction of the navicular and eversion of the heel.

In the flat-top talus, the posterior part of the trochlea is well rounded. Some of the deformity of the anterior part of the body and of the neck of the talus is acquired because in a persistent equinus deformity and limited ankle motion this portion of the talus never had the opportunity to mold in response to the normal physiologic stress of dorsiflexion. Overgrowth of the anterior body and failure to develop constriction of the neck of the talus contributes to the composite equinus deformity by impinging on the anterior lip of the tibia in dorsiflexion. Radiographs of the pathologic anatomy will vary in each case, depending on the patient's age and the severity of the deformity. Lastly, always keep in mind that radiographs show only the ossified portion of the tarsus.

REFERENCES

1. Beatson, T. R., and Pearson, J. R.: A method of assessing correction in clubfeet. Journal of Bone and Joint Surgery, *48B,* Feb. 1966.
2. Heywood, A. W. B.: The mechanics of the hindfoot in clubfoot as demonstrated radiographically. Journal of Bone and Joint Surgery, *46B:*102, 1964.
3. McKinnon, B., Evans, J., Browning, W. H.: Angle distortion in clubfoot roentgenograms. Paper presented at annual meeting of American Academy of Orthopaedic Surgeons, Atlanta, Ga., Feb. 7, 1980.
4. Simmons, G. W.: Analytical radiography of clubfeet. Journal of Bone and Joint Surgery, *59B,* Nov. 1977.
5. Templeton, A. W., McAlister, W. H., and Irwin, D. Z.: Standardization of terminology and evaluation of osseous relationships in congenitally abnormal feet. American Journal of Roentgenology, *93:*374-381, 1965.

6 | Nonoperative Treatment

The goal of treatment is to obtain a lasting correction—a plantigrade, pliable, cosmetically acceptable foot—in the shortest treatment time and with the least disruption of family life and the child's life. Patience, persistence, and many office or clinic visits are required to meet these goals, and therefore the family's cooperation and confidence are essential for a successful result.

INITIAL VISIT WITH PARENTS

Shortly after the baby is born, or on the first consultation, the orthopedist should explain to the parents the nature of the deformity, the course of treatment, the unpredictability of response to treatment, and the propensity for recurrent deformity. The distraught parents, particularly the child's mother, must be reassured that they are in no way responsible for the deformity. They invariably ask about the etiology and prognosis and must be told candidly that the etiology is still unknown. Inquisitive, intelligent parents appreciate a frank discussion of the various theories of etiology and a realistic prognosis. On the basis of clinical appearance at birth, I have been unable to determine, with any degree of consistent accuracy, the prognosis regarding the response to nonoperative treatment or the need for surgery to attain correction. A few extra minutes of the initial visit are time well spent in order to establish the good rapport so necessary in the management of this difficult problem. The confidence and cooperation of the parents must be established on the first visit. Since it is impossible to restore the clubfoot to complete normalcy, except in the mildest deformities, the family is forewarned that some varying degrees of residual abnormality, beyond the control of the surgeon, are to be expected.

The family should be reassured that, with their cooperation, prolonged treatment, and follow-up visits, the child will not be "a cripple" and will be able to walk, wear regular shoes, and enjoy a normal childhood and adult life, with some minor limitation. When the plan of treatment is outlined, the parents should be told realistically about all the problems that may arise. They should also be told that, in some cases, nonoperative treatment fails and surgery may be necessary. After a sympathetic discussion and explanation of the probable course of treatment, the parents may be more prepared to accept any eventuality. An informed family is a satisfied, cooperative family. It is advantageous to the parents if the orthopedist schedules their child for treatment on a day designated for clubfoot therapy in the office or in a special clinic. In this atmosphere, the parents gain comfort and reassurance by talking to other parents of children with clubfoot. They are also encouraged by the sight of older children who have recovered from the same disorder. This can also be accomplished by arranging appointments at a time when more than one child with clubfoot will be in the office, or by providing the distraught parents with the names of other clubfooted children in the community. Physicians must remember that they are dealing with the parents as well as the child with clubfoot.

METHODS OF NONOPERATIVE TREATMENT

Unlike the treatment of acute trauma and other orthopedic conditions, considerable time must elapse before a surgeon can profit and learn from his experience. I concur with McCauley,[14] who states: "Clubfeet tend to recur for at least 7 years." Fripp and Shaw[7] state: "At least 15 years elapse before any surgeon can assess the merit of the particular method he adopts, so that during his life in practice only two generations of patients come under his care. The opportunities to compare methods of primary treatment are limited and enthusiasm and pertinacity sometimes outweigh discernment." It is because of these factors, plus the infrequency of the condition, that a practicing orthopedist is denied the opportunity to evaluate enough of his results to change or modify his method of treatment.

There is general agreement that treatment should be started as soon as possible after birth, and that the initial treatment should be nonoperative. There are three different methods of nonoperative treatment: (1) manipulation and serial plaster of Paris casts, (2) stretching and adhesive strapping, and (3) Denis Browne splinting.

Proponents of each method have reported varying degrees of success. The method of treatment is an individual preference; the surgeon should use the method with which he or she is most comfortable and experienced. In this discussion, a method of management will be presented based on my personal experience, which evolved after analyzing the results and problems encountered with all three treatment methods. I am not implying that this is the only method of treatment; surgeons with more expertise in their favorite corrective procedure are capable of obtaining satisfactory results. The reader is referred to the references at the end of this chapter for details concerning the technique and results of the various methods of nonoperative treatment.[1-4,6-13,15,16]

The principles of treatment are based on the following concepts:

1.   The abnormal tarsal relationship is maintained by pathologic contractures of soft tissues.

2. The soft-tissue contractures must be stretched out in order to restore the normal tarsal relationships.

3. After a normal tarsal relationship is attained, correction must be maintained until the tarsal bones remold stable articular surfaces.

4. A recurrent deformity results from a failure to either attain a complete correction or maintain the correction.

NEONATAL EXAMINATION

Before embarking on treatment, one must inquire about unusual events during pregnancy and delivery and about other nonorthopedic congenital anomalies. It is especially important to inquire into the child's family history regarding clubfoot and neuromuscular skeletal conditions. A complete orthopedic examination is done to rule out other skeletal anomalies or neuromuscular conditions to make certain the foot deformity does not represent a local manifestation of a systemic or neuromuscular condition. The lumbosacral area is carefully examined for suspicious signs of meningomyelocele. Specifically, the examiner should look for conditions like arthrogryposis—Is the child a "floppy child" or robust and healthy? Is the child's cry normal or suspicious of a *Cri du Chat?* Is the child "funny looking"? Does the child move both legs normally? Are the hands normal? Does the child have a supernumerary thumb? Are finger- and toenails normal?

Unfortunately, it is not always possible to rule out a systemic syndrome. At birth, the child may appear to be afflicted with an idiopathic clubfoot which later is discovered to actually be part of a skeletal syndrome. The presence of diametrically opposite foot deformities, with a talipes equinovarus on one side and a contralateral talipes calcaneovalgus, is strong evidence of a nonidiopathic clubfoot deformity, especially meningomyelocele.

The size and flexibility of the foot may, at times, help to distinguish the idiopathic deformity. Usually, the longer and more flexible deformities, which are improved considerably with minimal stretching, suggest a neuromuscular or a readily correctable postural deformity. A critical, careful examination of the heel area is most helpful to distinguish the idiopathic deformity from an acquired or positional abnormality. In the idiopathic deformity, the posterior tuberosity is obscured, is difficult to palpate, and does not move up and down with dorsiflexion and plantar flexion; in addition, the usual skin creases in the region of the Achilles insertion are absent. It has been my experience that the presence of skin creases that are not as deep and as numerous as in the normal foot indicates an acquired deformity, as in a neurologic disorder or a myopathy. Unfortunately, it is not always possible to distinguish idiopathic from neuromuscular deformities.

Diagnosis of a nonidiopathic deformity does not alter the initial treatment. An accurate diagnosis, or a high degree of suspicion of a systemic condition at birth, is of value in order to give the family a more realistic prognosis and to outline the long-range treatment plan accordingly. This approach avoids the pitfalls, poor results, and complications of operative treatment, which occur more commonly after surgery for nonidiopathic deformities.

Neonatal Radiographs

Radiographs taken at birth confirm the clinical diagnosis and rule out osseous anomalies. During the course of treatment for clubfoot, many x-ray studies will be required. Therefore, to minimize x-ray exposure and because radiologic studies are of limited value at birth, they are not routinely done at the time of the initial examination. However, radiographs do provide a good clinical record, and I have no quarrel with those who feel they should be a routine part of the initial evaluation. Radiographs of the feet at birth are made when an osseous anomaly is suspected or the mother requests them in order "to make sure all the bones are present."

PRIMARY TREATMENT OF THE NEWBORN

Before treatment is undertaken, the infant's condition is explained to the parents and the treatment plan is outlined for them. Manipulation and plaster-cast immobilization are begun in the newborn nursery, as soon as possible. Except for some minor variations, the initial manipulation and cast treatment are essentially the same as that subsequently carried out in the course of treatment. The initial manipulation should be very gentle, using extreme care to avoid pressure over the dorsolateral aspect of the foot where the skin is often stretched out and quite thin. Therefore, the initial plaster cast requires more padding than subsequent ones. In some cases, considerable correction is possible after the initial manipulation. However, in the initial cast excessive correction should be avoided, especially in dorsiflexion, because circulatory and skin complications may result. The tips of all five toes must be clearly visible. If circulatory embarrassment evidenced by a persistent bluish discoloration of the toes is suspect, remove the plaster cast immediately and apply another one with the foot in less dorsiflexion. It is not unusual to notice a temporary slight bluish discoloration immediately after the manipulation, but the toes should "pink-up" immediately. The foot is kept elevated by propping sheets or towels under the leg. The nurses are instructed regarding the danger signs of circulatory impairment, and orders are left to remove the cast immediately if there is persistent bluish discoloration of the toes. Because the hospital stay is short, only one manipulation and casting usually is possible in the hospital. However, if, because of some maternal or concomitant pediatric problem, longer hospitalization is necessary, manipulation and cast treatments are repeated at more frequent intervals, while the child is in the hospital. The first cast is changed in the office at the earliest opportunity; this is usually 1 week after the patient is discharged.

MANIPULATION

Manipulation, before each cast is applied, is the most important part of nonoperative treatment. The objective is to stretch the soft-tissue contractures; the plaster of Paris cast serves to maintain the correction obtained by manipulation. Each successive manipulation gradually corrects more of the deformity until, hopefully, a full correction is obtained. During the manipulation, the surgeon should have a mental picture of the pathologic anatomy of the clubfoot and what he is trying to accomplish. The goals are to relocate the navicular in front of the talus and evert and dorsiflex the calcaneus.

The technique of manipulation is based on these concepts: equinus, varus, and adduction occur simultaneously and not as separate isolated components, and it is impossible to completely correct any one component of the deformity without, at the same time, eliminating the others. For these reasons, in the manipulation an attempt is made to correct all elements of the deformity simultaneously. This technique contrasts with the traditional method of "correcting adduction first, then varus, and lastly the equinus."[9]

Much emphasis has been placed on correcting the forefoot deformity first. In my experience, the adduction, varus, and equinus *of the forefoot* are usually readily corrected with manipulations. Elimination of the equinovarus of the heel and relocation of the navicular are the most difficult part of manipulation because it is difficult to manipulate the small inverted heel and exert pressure on the navicular. In addition, contractures that maintain these deformities are the most rigid.

All agree that manipulation should be "gentle." However, it must be pointed out that if it is "too gentle," it will be ineffective. Therefore, the manipulation should be gentle but yet strong enough to stretch the soft parts. Damage from manipulation treatment results from excessive dorsiflexion force, which can be easily applied on the long lever arm of the forefoot; it is difficult to apply excessive valgus force on the heel and the navicular.

The technique used to treat a right clubfoot deformity is as follows: an attempt is made to lengthen the Achilles and posterior contractures by exerting downward and everting pressure on the posterior tuberosity of the calcaneus; effective pressure can be applied with either the thumb or index finger. The medial contractures and the concavity of the medial border of the foot are stretched as follows: the left thumb exerts counterpressure over the dorsolateral prominence of the unexposed head and neck of the talus, while the right hand exerts forward traction on the medial border of the foot. If the navicular is palpable, direct forward pressure is exerted with the thumb over the region of the navicular. The forefoot deformity is usually loosened and corrected by the previously described maneuver. When the forefoot component of the deformity is more rigid or severe, the varus, adduction, and equinus are corrected by grasping the forefoot separately, while maintaining thumb pressure over the region of the sinus tarsi. Correction of the forefoot deformity is usually accomplished readily. This series of manipulations is repeated until it is felt that maximum loosening has been attained.

After the contractures have been softened, an attempt is made to correct all components of the deformity, simultaneously, as follows: the child's mother or physician's assistant stabilizes the thigh and knee while the surgeon grasps the foot with his right hand. Visualizing the deformity and what we are trying to accomplish, an attempt is made to realign the tarsus around the talus by correcting equinus, varus, and adduction simultaneously. The index finger exerts downward and valgus pressure on the heel, while the thumb exerts counterpressure on the head of the talus laterally; the palm of the hand abducts the forefoot and lengthens the medial border of the foot. The foot is then temporarily held in the corrected position and the manipulations repeated until it is felt that maximum correction has been achieved. In the bilateral deformity, the same procedure is carried out on the contralateral foot, and the cycle is repeated. Manipulation takes time; it cannot be hurried.

Invariably, the contractures loosen and the deformity improves following these maneuvers. The degree of correction depends on the rigidity and severity of the deformity. Small, rigid feet are the most difficult to improve with the manipulations.

PLASTER OF PARIS CASTING

Applying the Cast

Following adequate manipulation, an above-the-knee plaster cast is applied while the foot is held in maximum correction. Except for the initial plaster cast, which is applied in the newborn nursery, only one layer of Webril (thin cast padding) is used to pad the cast. The cast padding, like the plaster, should be applied smoothly, without wrinkles. The cast must fit snugly if it is to effectively maintain the correction achieved by manipulation. All too often, excessive cast padding is applied.

To apply the cast, I prefer to use 3-inch, fast-setting plaster. The first three turns of plaster are applied over the forefoot, directly on the cast padding and not over the fingers that are holding the toes. After the forefoot has been wrapped in plaster, the forefoot is grasped to hold the foot in dorsiflexion, while the ankle and heel are wrapped in plaster by oblique figure-of-eight turns over the instep. The borders of the plaster should not cross the dorsal aspect of the ankle joint transversely. Then while the plaster is setting, the foot is held in the position of maximum correction and the cast is molded around the heel to lock the calcaneus in the corrected position. Lateral force is exerted on the first metatarsal head.

With this technique, problems with cast pressure sores are avoided. Long leg casts with the knee flexed to a right angle are used routinely (Fig. 6-1). I have not been able to apply effective below-the-knee casts in infancy. In spite of the fact that only one layer of cast padding is applied with an above-knee cast, some children still kick their casts off. It is most difficult to apply and maintain a cast without slippage in children with significant equinus, extremely small inverted heel, chubby legs, short rigid feet, and considerable subcutaneous baby fat. Application of a plaster cast on these feet is "like trying to roll plaster over jello." Incorporating adhesive straps in the plaster has been tried and abandoned because of skin irritation. I have tried slipper casts and the wedging cast, as described by Kite,[10] but have not been able to duplicate his successful results.

Caring for the Cast

Mothers are advised to use self-sealing disposable diapers, and to cover the upper part of the cast and thigh with clear polyethylene wrap. These methods have been effective in keeping the cast clean and dry. Mothers are also taught to

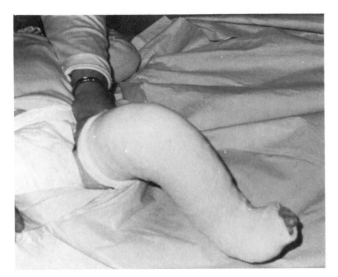

Fig. 6-1. Cast in infancy. A well-molded cast with the knee flexed avoids cast slippage and effectively maintains the correction attained by the manipulation. The protruding toes will disappear with cast slippage.

check the amount of toe protrusion from the cast; if the toes disappear, this is evidence of cast slippage. When cast slippage occurs, the mother removes the cast immediately and the child returns for another manipulation and cast treatment. With the knee flexed, quite frequently there will be some irritation in the posterior aspect of the upper thigh. This can be avoided by elevating the leg.

Removing the Cast

The child's mother removes the plaster cast just before she brings the child to the physician's office for remanipulation and cast immobilization. The plaster cast should not be removed the night before. In the past, the correction invariably was lost and the deformity promptly recurred overnight. When this technique is used, the mother is instructed to place the child in a bathinette to soak the cast. While in the water, the cast is softened by repeated squeezing, so that the plaster can be unwound for removal. Leaving several folds of the plaster at the end of the roll to initiate the process facilitates the unwinding. The mother's proficiency improves with experience. This method provides an opportunity to bathe the child and avoids the psychologic trauma, to both mother and child, of the electric cast cutter, especially with a snug cast. Finally, the short period of exposure is beneficial for skin care. This method of removal is used in the infant. The electric cast cutter is preferable in the older child with a thicker cast, and to remove a walking cast.

Frequency of Manipulations

It is desirable to remanipulate and change casts as frequently as possible—every few days would be ideal. However, practically it has been impossible to do this more frequently than once a week. The casts are changed at weekly intervals for the first 6 to 8 weeks. During this period, the correction is most dramatic. Thereafter, the casts are changed less frequently. Treatment is continued as long as further correction is achieved with serial manipulations.

EVALUATION AT 2 TO 3 MONTHS OF AGE

After 2 to 3 months of treatment, the correction is critically evaluated both radiologically and clinically to assess the response to and plan the future course of treatment. Even though most of the anlagen of the calcaneus and talus are not ossified at 2 to 3 months of age, there is sufficient ossification for useful radiologic evaluation (Fig. 6-2). In the uncorrected foot, the calcaneus shows no dorsiflexion in the stress dorsiflexion lateral view—the anterior ends of the talus and calcaneus may show apparent overlap. At this age, clinical examination may reveal an apparent correction because the equinus deformity of the hindfoot is camouflaged by dorsiflexion of the forefoot, and a laterally shifted heel pad is mistaken as a correction of the inverted calcaneus. Such a "spurious correction" is recognized by focusing attention on the posterior tuberosity of the calcaneus, or by comparison with the normal heel in the unilateral deformity. In the corrected foot, the posterior tuberosity can both be seen and palpated, moving downward as the foot is dorsiflexed. In the spurious correction, the posterior tuberosity is small, inverted, difficult to palpate, and vertical motion is limited.

Utilizing both the radiologic and the clinical examination, the correction and the response to treatment can be evaluated quite accurately at this age. Evaluation between 2 and 3 months of age is important, because if a complete correction has not been attained after 2 to 3 months of treatment the deformity usually will not respond to nonoperative treatment. Through the years, this observation has been quite accurate for determining prognosis regarding response to treatment. On the basis of this evaluation, a decision is made either to continue nonoperative treatment or plan for future surgical correction. One should not get the impression that the surgical course is readily accepted; on the contrary, every effort is made to avoid surgery. I feel that correction by nonoperative methods is the treatment of choice, when possible.

If the evaluation at this stage of treatment reveals the deformity has improved but is not necessarily a complete correction, manipulations and cast treatment are not discontinued. They are continued as long as there is evidence of improvement and the response to manipulations is satisfactory.

MANAGEMENT

Successful Nonoperative Treatment

When the evaluation at 2 to 3 months shows a satisfactory correction, the foot is held in an overcorrected position by a series of plaster casts for a total of

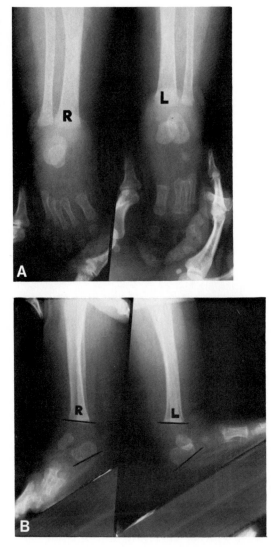

Fig. 6-2. Bilateral clubfeet at 3 months. *(A)*, After 3 months of serial manipulations and plaster, only the left foot showed clinical evidence of correction. This was corroborated by the radiographic evaluation. Enough ossification is present to assess hindfoot divergence. Note the superimposition of the calcaneus and talus on the right, whereas the left foot shows good divergence of the long axes of the bones. *(B),* At 3 months of age the radiologic evaluation revealed persistent equinus of the calcaneus. The left foot responded to nonoperative treatment, whereas the right foot eventually required surgical correction. This case illustrates: the reliability of radiologic assessment to evaluate the correction and response to treatment; if a correction is not obtained after several months of treatment, surgery is usually necessary to correct the deformity; and the unpredictability of response to treatment in bilateral clubfeet, with invariably one side being more resistant than the other.

6 to 8 months. The overcorrected position is really one of maximum correction because it is difficult to overcorrect an idiopathic clubfoot with nonoperative treatment. The casts are changed periodically, commensurate with "spurts" in growth. The plaster must be snug and well-molded to lock the heel in the dorsiflexed position. I prefer to use above-knee casts; a below-knee cast is used only after the child has lost his "baby fat," the foot and leg have grown, and I feel confident there is no danger of losing the correction in plaster.

After 6 to 8 months of plaster immobilization, a 10-inch Denis Browne (D-B) bar with attached tarsopronator shoes is used to maintain correction (Fig. 6-3). The D-B bar is worn for 24 hours a day. It is removed for exercise and passive stretching for only a few minutes when the baby is bathed, fed, or his

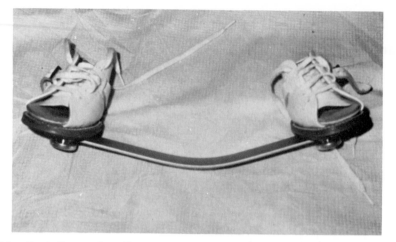

Fig. 6-3.   Denis Browne bar. Open-toe tarsopronator shoes are attached to a D-B bar 20 to 25 cm long in 10° of external rotation. The bar is slightly concave toward the patient.

diaper is changed. These short periods of exercise and activity are desirable and beneficial in preventing further disuse atrophy.

The child is checked at frequent intervals to make certain the correction is maintained and instructions are being followed. The mother is forewarned of the possibility of recurrent deformity; she is advised to look for heel-cord shortening. The first visible sign of loss of correction is the recurrence of equinus. The child's mother usually notices that it is difficult to get the foot into the shoe because of a "tight heel cord." In some cases, a temporary mild shortening of the heel cord develops during a growth spurt. This temporary shortening usually responds to a short course of manipulation and immobilization in plaster. However, if a significant equinovarus deformity fails to respond to treatment and the deformity increases, this occurrence is suspicious of a resistant foot that will require surgical correction. When the child approaches the walking stage, he should not be discouraged to walk; on the contrary, he should be encouraged to do so. Weight bearing and walking with tarsopronator shoes provide a physiologic stimulus for tarsal remolding, stretch the heel cord, and prevent further disuse atrophy. The walking child continues to use a D-B bar at naptime and during the night for several years.

Even though clinical and x-ray evaluations show apparent satisfactory correction, the family is told that the deformity may still recur until age 7. For this reason, it is necessary to follow instructions and return for periodic reevaluations.

Borderline Corrections

Occasionally, in the 6- to 12-month age group, there are borderline corrections. That is, the clubfoot is not completely corrected by rigid critical radiologic assessment; clinically, the feet are plantigrade and have no significant heel varus; dorsiflexion, while limited, is possible to above the right angle; and, most important, there is no evidence of increasing deformity. In these cases, nonoperative treatment is continued. Every attempt should be made to maintain the correction with bivalved corrective casts at night and at naptime, corrective walking shoes, and passive stretching exercises. During this time, the child can exercise his leg muscles, thereby avoiding further disuse atrophy and weakness. Surgical correction can be done later if the correction is lost and the deformity recurs.

Braces and Splints

In my experience, corrective braces, with and without spring attachments, used at night or during the day have been unsuccessful in correcting a deformity or preventing an increasing deformity of an incompletely corrected foot. I have found that the most effective method of maintaining the desired position at night is the use of a well-molded snug fitting bivalved cast. The disadvantage of plastic orthoses is that it is difficult to make a splint that will correct the combination of equinus, varus, and adduction, and hold the foot as firmly as a well-molded, snug bivalved cast (Fig. 6-4).

After a complete correction is attained it is essential to maintain the correction at night. A Denis Browne bar is used in small children; in the older child, a bivalved cast is used.

Treatment with Denis Browne (D-B) Splint. The D-B splint[4,5] consists of two foot pieces connected by a cross bar. Each foot is strapped into a foot piece. The rationale of this method depends upon the active kicking movement of each leg, exerting a corrective force on its counterpart (Fig. 6-5). When this method was first reported, there were many advocates; but the number of surgeons in the United States who use this method is dwindling. In earlier years, I repeatedly tried this method alone or in combination with manipulation and cast immobilization, but abandoned it because of the high incidence of failures and problems encountered with skin irritation. Fripp and Shaw[7] reported a high incidence of failures using the DB splint. In my experience, the splint was successful in the long flexible type of deformity but I found it impossible to apply the splint on small rigid feet with a small inverted heel and severe deformity. In addition to the high rate of failure, this method is prone to cause problems with skin irritation; often this was the reason the method had to be discontinued.

Treatment with Adhesive Strapping. In this method, multiple long straps of adhesive tape are wrapped around the foot in the direction of correction and extended over the lower thigh with the knee in 90° of flexion. The principle of this method depends on the child's knee motion to apply an eversion corrective force on the foot (Fig. 6-6). Advocates of this method maintain that the child's normal activity provides a dynamic correction; however, it is not generally used at the present time. Most proponents of the method are from the English school of orthopaedics.[3,7] Lusskin[12] and Lusskin[13] in the United States have been enthusiastic with this method. The method requires repeated and frequent rebandaging and reinforcements over the initial adhesive strapping. My limited experience with

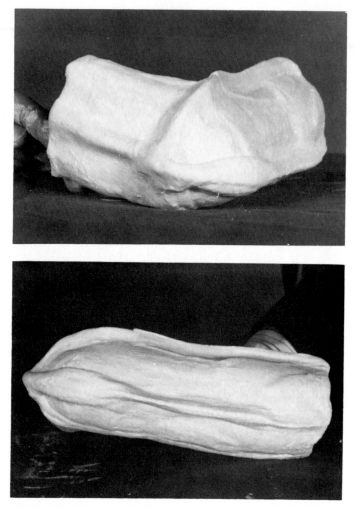

Fig. 6-4.   Plaster splint for use at night and naptime. A plaster splint will maintain the foot in the maximum overcorrected position more effectively and is more economical than a plastic orthosis. The plaster is reinforced by longitudinal strips of plaster over the edges and the middle of the cast. These "ropes" of plaster serve as "I beams" that make the plaster more durable to withstand the activity of children.

the method has been unsuccessful due primarily to the problems with skin irritation and blistering; invariably the treatment had to be discontinued because of the skin abrasions.

RESULTS OF NONOPERATIVE TREATMENT

The term relapsed foot infers that the deformity recurred after prior correction. Brockman[4] is of the opinion that the so-called relapsed foot really represents an

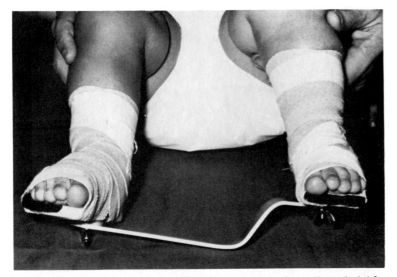

Fig. 6-5. Denis Browne splint modified for treatment of a unilateral clubfoot.

increasing recurrent deformity of an incomplete correction. Retrospective, close scrutiny of the radiographs in these cases often reveals that in fact the foot was not completely corrected. This statement is applicable primarily to the idiopathic clubfoot.

Many authors have written on the high incidence of failures and *relapse?* following the three basic methods of nonoperative treatment. Often, this was a combination of two methods or, in some series, neonatal percutaneous tenotomy of the achilles tendon was considered part of nonoperative management. The success rate of these series ranged from a low of 19 percent to a high of 90 percent.[1-5,7-12,16,17,18-20] Kite[11] reported 90 percent success with his method of manipulation and casting, which he continues for years if necessary. Fripp and Shaw[8] treated 105 feet with the Denis Browne splints and corrected 19 percent, whereas 71 percent of 96 treated by manipulation and stretching were corrected. Only 20 feet were treated by manipulation and serial plaster of Paris casts; all these required surgery. Dangelmajor[7] in a review of 200 successive unselected cases reported 40 percent were corrected with nonoperative treatment; the average total time under active care to achieve the final result was 4 years. Blockey and Smith[3] reviewed 186 feet treated with nonoperative treatment, which included a combination of adhesive splinting, Denis Browne splint, manipulation under anesthesia, and D-B bar. In this series of 186 feet, 121 relapsed; the deformity recurred in the first year in 8, between 1 and 2 years in 48, and between 2 and 3 years in 65.

Review of my experience with patients treated from birth with a follow-up of 7 years revealed 35 percent were successfully treated with nonoperative management. The milder deformities, which were completely corrected after 2 to 3 months of treatment, tended to stay corrected. The correction present at age 7 is usually maintained in the idiopathic deformity; this is not applicable to the nonidiopathic clubfoot. For the above reason, McCauley[15] stated that when a clubfoot appears

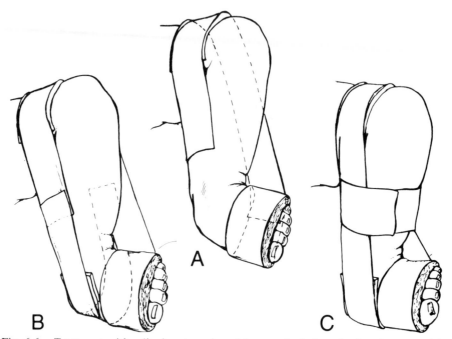

Fig. 6-6.   Treatment with adhesive strapping. After manipulation, the foot is strapped in the position of maximum correction. The mother is instructed how to stretch the foot. Frequent medical supervision is necessary with this method of treatment. More strapping is placed over the original to increase correction. *(A),* A strip of adhesive orthopaedic felt is placed around the forefoot and a similar piece above the knee. Adhesive strapping is then applied; beginning laterally, it passes over the dorsum, then the sole of the foot, up the lateral side of the leg, over the knee, and down the medial side to hold the foot dorsiflexed and everted. *(B),* A third strip of orthopaedic felt is placed around the heel, and adhesive tape is passed under the heel from the medial to the lateral side of the leg to maintain eversion and encourage dorsiflexion of the calcaneus. *(C),* Slack or bowstringing of the adhesive is taken up by another piece of adhesive tape applied around the leg. (Fripp, A. T., and Shaw, N. E.: Clubfoot. E. and S. Livingstone, Edinburgh and London, 1967.)

corrected at 6 months of age, the parents are told "one-fourteenth of the treatment time has been completed." Some of the more severe deformities required repeated courses of manipulation with serial plaster immobilization and the prolonged protection of night splints.

The long-term follow-up revealed many feet appeared to be corrected for a while; however, they later developed a recurrent deformity and required surgical correction, up to the age of 7 years (Fig. 6-7). Some of the feet treated without surgery were satisfactory acceptable corrections, even though slightly incomplete, providing the correction was maintained without evidence of increasing deformity. A plantigrade foot with minimal varus and slight limitation of dorsiflexion without callosities can be a serviceable acceptable correction, providing there is no evidence of increasing deformity.

Increasing deformity in the clubfoot is comparable to scoliosis; a minimal,

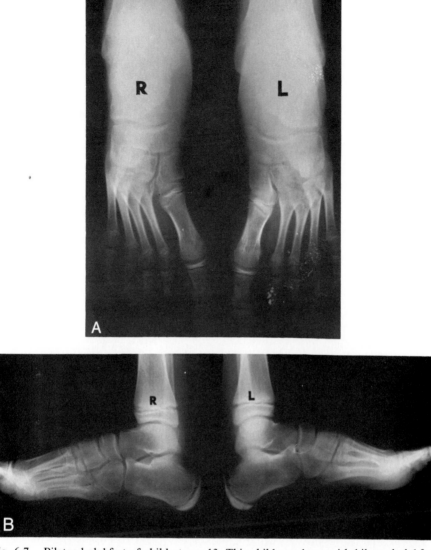

Fig. 6-7. Bilateral clubfeet of child at age 13. This child was born with bilateral clubfeet that were treated from birth. Satisfactory correction was obtained bilaterally after 6 months of serial manipulation and plaster, followed by D-B bar application. At 5 years of age, the child developed a mild contracture of the right heel cord. Despite serial manipulations and casts followed by night splints, the equinovarus deformity became progressively worse. Eventually the child was unable to get his right foot into a shoe or the night splint. At age seven, a soft tissue release and a Steindler stripping were necessary to correct the increasing deformity of the right foot. Excellent correction was maintained on the left side without any operative intervention. This case shows the tendency of the deformity to recur after apparent correction up to the age of seven. The case also demonstrates that in bilateral deformities one foot is usually more resistant to treatment than the other. Fig. 6-7(A), Note that in the right foot, which required surgical correction, there is less hindfoot divergence and a slight metatarsus adductus. (B), The talus in the right foot shows an abnormal shape of the anterior trochlea and less constriction of the neck. Dorsiflexion on the right side is slightly limited in comparison with the left. The left foot is almost normal.

continued increasing deformity by increments of 1° to 2° eventually becomes an unacceptable result functionally and cosmetically. Increasing deformity should be distinguished from temporary mild shortening of the heel cord associated with growth spurts; this occurrence is not unusual.

MANAGEMENT OF THE RESISTANT FOOT

The author concurs with McCauley[15] that if complete correction has not been attained after 2 to 3 months of adequate treatment, in most cases surgical correction will be necessary. A foot is considered resistant when the deformity shows no evidence of further improvement with manipulations, and the radiographic and clinical examinations confirm the persistence of equinovarus deformity. In these cases, manipulation treatment has failed to overcome the soft-tissue contractures that are preventing reduction of the navicular and the calcaneus to their normal relationship with the talus. In my experience, continuation of manipulation and nonoperative treatment for the resistant foot has been nonproductive and, in addition, can cause iatrogenic problems (compression changes of the talus or rockerbottom deformity). When a diagnosis of resistant clubfoot is made, manipulation and immobilization treatments are discontinued; at this time, a D-B bar is used, if possible, or a tendo Achillis lengthening is done when necessary.

Use of the D-B bar or preliminary achilles lengthening has avoided rockerbottom deformity attributable to the discontinuation of nonproductive persistent manipulations in the resistant foot. With this regimen of treatment, less fibrosis and deformity of the talus have been noticed at surgery. This management of the resistant foot avoids repeated office visits, unproductive treatment, iatrogenic problems, and muscle atrophy, which develop with prolonged manipulations and immobilization.

Denis Browne (D-B) Bar as a Holding Splint

A D-B bar with attached open-toe tarsopronator shoes is used for the "spurious" correction. The apparatus is worn 24 hours a day and removed for passive stretching. The D-B bar serves as a holding device to prevent increasing deformity and affords an opportunity for exercise while awaiting definitive corrective surgery that is done when the child is around 1 year old. Occasionally, in spite of this management, because of increasing equinus, the mother may be unable to apply the shoe. In this situation, a short course of weekly manipulations has been usually successful in eliminating the increased equinus and resumption of the use of the D-B bar, while awaiting surgical correction (Figs. 6-8 and 6-9).

Preliminary Tendo-Achillis Lengthening (TAL)

Some recalcitrant feet have persistent, very severe equinovarus deformities even after several months of manipulation and cast treatment. These are the small,

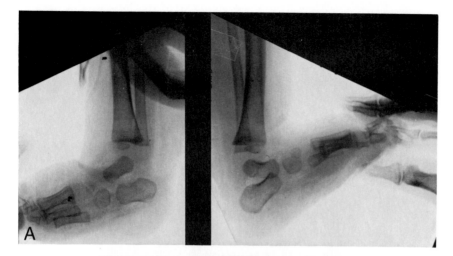

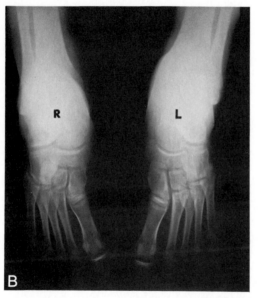

Fig. 6-8.   Use of a D-B bar as a holding device for the resistant foot. This child with a right clubfoot was seen for the first time at 4 months. Manipulations and serial casting had been initiated in the nursery. The clinical examination at this time showed typical findings of a resistant uncorrected deformity. Lateral radiographs confirmed the clinical diagnosis [Fig. 6-8*(A)*]. At 4 months of age manipulations were discontinued, the mother was instructed in passive stretching exercises, and a D-B bar was used as a holding splint while awaiting surgical correction. A one-stage soft tissue release was done at 11 months. Discontinuation of manipulations and plaster minimized disuse atrophy and avoided months of unproductive office visits and manipulations, as well as fibrosis and iatrogenic changes of the talus. The radiographs at skeletal maturity show satisfactory results with this management [Fig. 6-8*(B)*]. *(A)*, Radiograph at 4 months of age. Comparison dorsiflexion lateral views show no dorsiflexion of the calcaneus in the right foot (on the left). *(B)*, Radiograph at 15 years shows satisfactory tarsal relationship in comparison with the normal left foot.

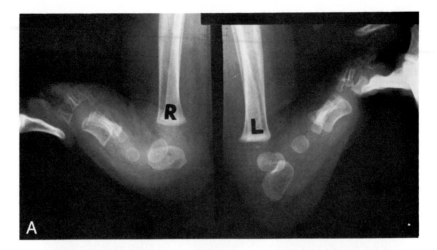

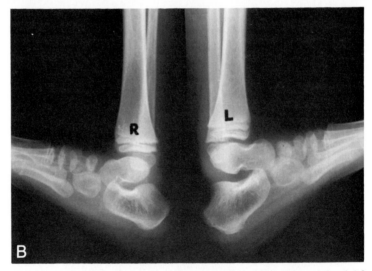

Fig. 6-9.   Management of rocker-bottom deformity. This child with a right clubfoot developed a rocker-bottom deformity after three and one-half months of treatment with manipulation and plaster. Continuation of manipulations in a rocker-bottom is futile, because slight upward pressure causes a breach at the hypermobile tarsometatarsal level [Fig. 6-9(A)]. An attempt was made to correct the rocker-bottom by immobilizing the foot in equinus for several weeks and then resuming dorsiflexion of the foot. Three serial attempts to correct the rocker-bottom by this maneuver were unsuccessful; deformity recurred each time dorsiflexion was attempted. Manipulations and casting were discontinued, and a D-B bar was used until 14 months of age, at which time a one-stage posteromedial release was done. This case illustrates the futility of continuation of manipulations and plaster in children that develop a rocker-bottom.

Fig. 6-9.   *(A),* Radiograph at 4 months. Comparison views show typical rocker-bottom of right foot with slight upward pressure on the forefoot. *(B),* At 8 years of age.

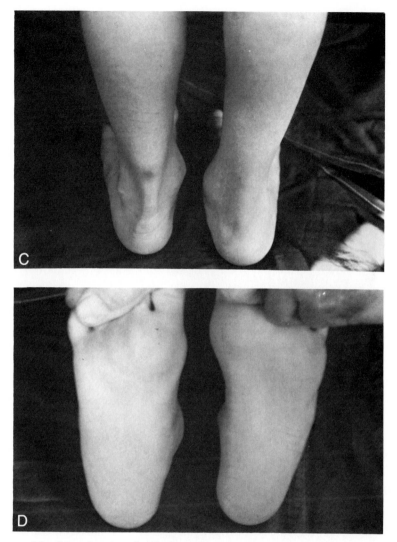

Fig. 6-9.   *(continued) (C)*, Rear view, standing. *(D)*, Plantar view.

rigid feet, with small, markedly inverted and plantar flexed heels that often have a deep cleft above the heel or in the plantar surface. These feet are the most difficult to manipulate and keep in effective plaster casts. The severe equinus precludes the use of a D-B bar because it is impossible to put a shoe on the foot. In these deformities, a preliminary TAL is done at the musculotendinous junction. Lengthening the Achilles proximally serves to facilitate the one-stage posteromedial release by avoiding postoperative scarring just above the ankle. Postoperatively, the child is treated with manipulations and casts for 6 weeks, and the D-B bar is then used while awaiting definitive surgery (Fig. 6-10). Infrequently, the equinus has been so severe that after the TAL the foot had to be immobilized in slight equinus because the skin blanched in dorsiflexion due to marked shortening of the neurovascular bundle. On very rare occasions, preliminary achilles lengthening has produced correction of one side in a bilateral deformity.

Preliminary TAL has also been carried out in a small series of patients that were seen for the first time at age 4 to 7 months (Fig. 6-11). This group includes the most severe deformities, with persistent severe equinus in spite of prior adequate treatment. The rationale of preliminary TAL in this group is to minimize the equinus deformity of the ankle joint and allow more of the talus to enter the mortise, thus preventing further overgrowth of the anterior portion of the trochlea and the neck of the talus while awaiting definitive surgery. Partial correction at this age facilitates surgery and permits more dorsiflexion with the subsequent one-stage release operation; an added advantage is that the increased ankle motion prevents further disuse atrophy and stretches the contracted skin. After the Achilles lengthening, the Denis Browne bar is used as a holding device.

(continued on page 107)

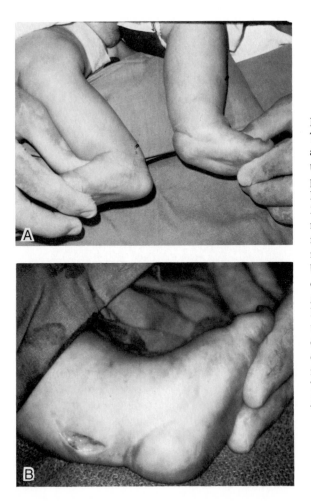

Fig. 6-10. Preliminary TAL. This case illustrates the management of extremely recalcitrant deformed feet with early preliminary TAL proximally. Fig. 6-10(A). Left clubfoot at 3 months of age following manipulation and plaster treatment which was started in the nursery. The use of the D-B bar was impossible, because equinus deformity precluded getting the foot into a shoe. Note the small, inverted heel with a deep cleft above the calcaneus. Fig. 6-10(B). Intraoperative photograph shows increased dorsiflexion after TAL at the musculotendinous junction at 3 months of age.

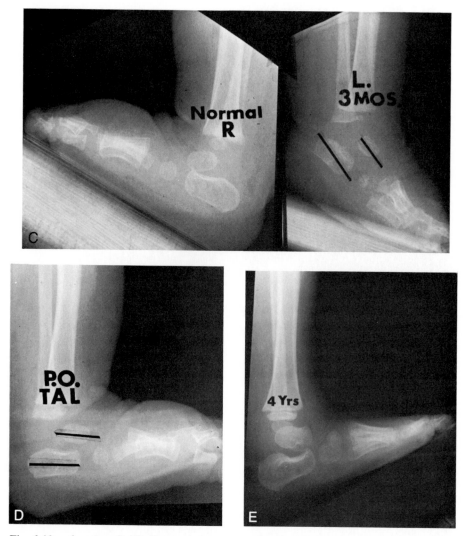

Fig. 6-10. *(continued) (C),* Comparison preoperative dorsiflexion lateral radiograph shows severe equinus with parallelism of the calcaneus and talus of the left foot. *(D),* Intraoperative lateral view after TAL shows dorsiflexion to a right angle. However, note that the relationship between the calcaneus and talus is unchanged—the two bones are still parallel to one another. The increased dorsiflexion occurred only in the ankle joint, as more of the talus entered the mortise. *(E),* A one-stage release with internal fixation was done at 1 year of age. Radiograph *E* shows correction at 4 years of age.

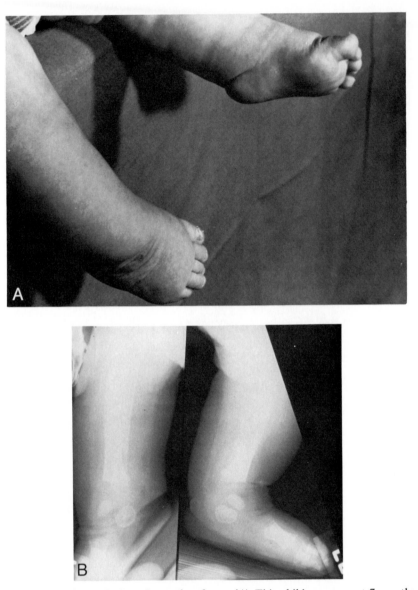

Fig. 6-11.   Preliminary TAL at 7 months of age. *(A),* This child was seen at 7 months of age with severe bilateral clubfoot deformities that had failed to respond to manipulation and plaster immobilization. Maintenance of casts in children having these severe equinovarus deformities with considerable baby fat and small, chubby feet is very difficult. *(B),* Radiographs at 7 months of age prior to bilateral preliminary TAL. After TAL was performed, the feet were maintained in the corrected position in plaster for 6 weeks, following which a D-B bar was used while awaiting definitive surgery.

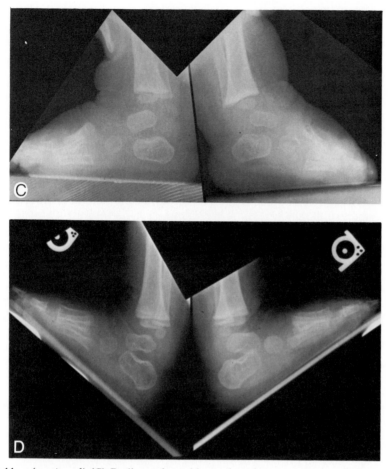

Fig. 6-11. *(continued) (C),* Radiographs at 14 months prior to one-stage soft tissue release. Surgery after a prior preliminary TAL was facilitated because the deformity was less severe; the contracted skin was stretched. It was easier to maintain the surgical correction in plaster with less baby fat and a larger foot. *(D),* Radiographs at four and one-half years of age show good correction.

My experiences with posterior release (TAL, tibiotalar, and subtalar capsulotomies) at an early age were disappointing. Furthermore, the postsurgical scarring in the area made subsequent surgery much more difficult. For these reasons, early posterior release was abandoned in favor of a high preliminary TAL when severe equinus made use of the D-B bar impossible, while waiting until the child was old enough for a complete soft-tissue release.

REFERENCES

1. Beatson, T. R.: A method of assessing correction in clubfeet. Journal of Bone and Joint Surgery, *48B:*38, 1966.

2. Bertelsen, A.: Treatment of congenital clubfoot. Journal of Bone and Joint Surgery, *39B:*599, 1957.

3. Blockey, M. J., and Smith, M. G. H.: The treatment of congenital clubfoot. Journal of Bone and Joint Surgery, *48B:*660, 1966.

4. Brockman, E. P.: Congenital clubfoot. John Wright and Sons, Bristol, 1930.

5. Browne, D.: Talipes equinovarus. Lancet, *2:*969, 1934.

6. Browne, D.: Splinting for controlled movement. Clinical Orthopaedics, *8:*91, 1956.

7. Dangelmajor, R. C.: A review of 200 clubfeet. Bulletin of the Hospital for Special Surgery, *4:*38, 1961.

8. Fripp, A. T., and Shaw, N. E.: Clubfoot. E. and S. Livingstone, Edinburgh and London, 1967.

9. Jansen, K.: Treatment of congenital clubfoot. Journal of Bone and Joint Surgery, *39B:*599, 1957.

10. Kite, H. J.: Principles involved in treatment of clubfoot. Journal of Bone and Joint Surgery, *2:*595, 1939.

11. Kite, H. J.: Non-operative treatment of congenital clubfoot. Clinical Orthopedics and Related Research, *84:*29, 1972.

12. Lovell, W. W., and Hancock, C. I.: Treatment of congenital talipes equinovarus. Clinical Orthopedics and Related Research, *70:*79, 1970.

13. Lusskin, R.: Neonatal treatment of congenital clubfoot by dynamic adhesive strapping. American Academy of Orthopedic Surgery Sound Slide Program No. 379.

14. Lusskin, R.: Neonatal therapy for congenital clubfoot. Interclinic Information Bulletin, *9:*1-7, New York University J. July, 1972.

15. McCauley, J. C.: The history of conservative and surgical methods of clubfoot treatment. Clinical Orthopaedics and Related Research, *84:*25, 1972.

16. Ponsetti, I. V., and Smolley, E. M.: Congenital clubfoot: The results of treatment. Journal of Bone and Joint Surgery, *45A:*261, 1963.

17. Shaw, N. E.: The early management of clubfoot. Clinical Orthopaedics and Research, *84:*38, 1972.

18. Wynne-Davies, R.: Review of eighty-four cases after completion of treatment. Journal of Bone and Joint Surgery, *46B:*38, 1964.

7 | Operative Treatment

REVIEW OF OPERATIVE TECHNIQUES

Many methods have been recommended for the surgical correction of resistant clubfoot. These have included, soft tissue release, tendon transfers, and bony operations. Some procedures are piecemeal operations intended to correct one specific component of the deformity, and many one- and two-stage operations have been described to correct all components of the deformity. The rationale for each method is based on varying concepts of the basic pathology. In addition, opinions differ regarding the optimum age for surgery. The reader is referred to the references for details of the respective techniques.[1-6,9,14,15,17,19,22,26,27,31,35,37,38]

The innumerable published articles on the surgical treatment of clubfeet is ample evidence that many cases fail to respond to nonoperative management.[2,3,46] And, the numerous operative methods described reveal that there is no concensus regarding the method of surgical correction.

McCauley[27] recommended surgical treatment "when it is established that dorsiflexion of the talus and calcaneus cannot be produced by stretching force, and this can be determined only by x-ray examination and not by clinical appearance." In his opinion, the optimum age for soft-tissue release was between 3½ and 5 years of age. He recommended a medial release with lengthening of the tibialis posterior; a TAL and posterior capsulotomies are done as a second-stage operation 6 to 8 weeks later, when necessary. McCauley recommended that one should correct as much as the contracted skin allows—"skin tension decides the amount of correction." He relied on plaster casts to maintain the surgical correction.

Attenborough[1] described an operation based on the rationale that the "fundamental deformity in severe clubfeet is the fixed plantar flexion of the talus." His method of surgical correction consists of a posterior capsulotomy and lengthening of the tendo achilles, sectioning the tibialis posterior, the flexor hallucis longus, and the flexor digitorum longus. After surgery the foot is held in maximum dorsiflexion for 6 weeks in a plaster cast. After the cast is removed, a "Denis-Browne splint is used for a few months, or until the child can maintain correction with its own muscles." He reported on a series of 22 operations, with a surgical age of 2 to 4 months and a follow-up of 6 months to 4 years. He noted that "all the divided tendons appear to function normally within a few months."

Main and his coworkers[25] reviewed 77 Attenborough operations. In 39 feet of their series, the operation was modified to include a medial release. Postoperatively, most cases were treated with adhesive strapping, and after the patients were discharged from the hospital, the strapping was changed and reinforced, as necessary, by physiotherapists. In a few cases, a plaster or Paris cast was used for about 5 days followed by strapping. The results were "analyzed after one operation (first assessment) and after subsequent operation (second assessment) on the basis of clinical appraisal." One-half of the patients achieved a satisfactory result after the first operation and 15 unsuccessful results were made satisfactory by further surgery. The subsequent operations included eight soft-tissue procedures and a combination of soft tissue and bony operations in the other seven feet. The conclusions from these data were: the posteromedial release has a slight advantage over the posterior release operation; the best results were obtained with early surgery (before 6 to 8 weeks of age); and if surgery was done after 6 to 8 weeks, the talonavicular joint should also be released.

Goldner[17] described an operation based on the concept that the major deformity is an "internal rotation of the talus in the ankle joint, the forefoot is adducted and inverted, and the calcaneus moves with the talus." Based on this rationale, his method of surgical correction concentrates on releasing the ankle ligaments in order to reposition the talus in the mortise. When necessary, subsequent soft-tissue operations and tendon transfers or bony procedures are carried out. Bleck[4] has reported satisfactory results with this technique. Carroll's[8] approach is just the opposite of Goldner's. In his opinion, the talus is rotated laterally in the ankle mortise, therefore his surgical approach is directed towards derotating the talus in the opposite direction.

Wagner and Butterfield[43] described a two-stage medial and posterior release (PMR). In the first stage, a partial medial release with excision of a segment of posterior tibial tendon is done and the tuberosity of the navicular, when prominent, is resected. If necessary, 3 weeks later, posterior capsulotomy and TAL are carried out.

Hadidi[19] has described a one-stage operation aimed at correcting all components of the deformity and maintaining the correction by dorsolateral transfer of the tibialis posterior tendon. The operation includes: a medial plantar dissection of the contractures; release of the abductor hallucis at its insertion; transfer of the tibialis posterior to the dorsal aspect of the foot, subcutaneously around the medial malleolus and not anteriorly through the interosseous space; and a posterior release. The operative age is between 4 and 6 months.

Heyman's tarsometatarsal release is done in cases in which forefoot adduction recurred after the one-stage operation.

Bost[5] described a medial plantar and subtalar soft-tissue release. He emphasized the importance of dividing the master knot of Henry and adequate exposure to release the plantar contractures. When full correction was not possible, the deformity was gradually corrected after wound healing, either by repeated cast changes or by wedging casts. He warned about problems with wound healing and the danger of overcorrection.

Evan's[12] operation is based on the rationale that the major deformity is in the midtarsal joint. On the basis of this concept, a medial release is done and the calcaneocuboid joint is fused in order to stablize the correction and shorten the convex lateral column of the foot.

Results of Surgical Treatment

Dangelmajor[10] reviewed 200 unselected cases of clubfeet and found that 60 percent of these cases required soft tissue or bony surgery. An average of 2.7 operations per foot were performed on the 109 patients who were found to require surgery. Dangelmajor defined "active care" as the total amount of time necessary under active treatment to achieve the final result. This included application of casts, both corrective and postoperative, bracing and surgery. It did not, however, include the use of night splints.

The active treatment time for the patients who required surgery was 8 years and 4 months. Twenty-four (12 percent) of the 200 patients were eventually treated with a triple arthrodesis. He reported good results in 45 percent of the cases treated with surgery. Kuhlman and Bell[22] evaluated the operative procedures carried out on 53 patients with resistant congenital clubfeet. These 53 patients required a total of 154 operations (2.9 operations per patient), with 31 percent satisfactory results. The average age of the patient at the time of soft-tissue surgery was 4½ years; the average age at the time of bony surgery was 9 years. They noted that "in spite of good initial correction, recurrence was common between the first and second years postoperative." Eighteen of the 53 patients required bony operations, these included 12 triple arthrodeses, one ankle fusion, one astragalectomy, and two derotational osteotomies of the tibia.

My personal experience with medial release, posterior release, two-stage procedures, and rotational osteotomies were comparable to those reported by both Dangelmajor and Kuhlman. There was a high incidence of problems with wound healing in both the one- and two-stage soft-tissue operations; a small percent of satisfactory results were attained in some of the milder deformities.

The past objections to early soft-tissue operations, done to attain a complete operation, were: a high incidence of recurrent deformity; a high percentage of problems with wound healing; postoperative stiffness; and as extensive soft-tissue surgery was difficult in the small deformed foot, it was therefore contraindicated until the child was 3 to 4 years old. For these reasons, the resistant uncorrected foot was usually treated with piecemeal operations; years of manipulations, plaster casts, and braces; and special shoes. The standard accepted recommendation was to return at "maturity for a triple arthrodesis."

ONE-STAGE POSTEROMEDIAL RELEASE (PMR) WITH INTERNAL FIXATION

Dissatisfaction with the results of the various piecemeal operations and two-stage procedures provided the incentive to develop a one-stage PMR with internal fixation. I have used the method, to be described, on 273 feet.[39-42] My training was under the tutelage of McCauley and Wagner; therefore, the technique evolved from their methods of surgical correction. However, after my interest in clubfoot increased, a review of the literature revealed that the procedure to be described is essentially a modification of others described by Phelps[28] in 1891, by Codvilla[9] in 1906, by Brockman[6] in 1937, and by Bost[5] in 1960.

The operation is based on the following concepts:

1. The deformity is due to a congenital subluxation of the talocalcaneonavicular joint.

2. Correction of the abnormal tarsal relationship is prevented by rigid pathologic soft-tissue contractures.

3. There are two prerequisites for a lasting correction: complete correction must be obtained, and the surgical correction must be maintained while tarsal bones remold to form stable articular surfaces.

4. It is impossible to completely correct any one component of deformity without simultaneously eliminating the others.

The objectives of treatment are to obtain a lasting correction, i.e., a pliable, plantigrade, cosmetically acceptable foot, in one operation with minimal risk and a relatively short treatment time.

Indications.   The operation is recommended for resistant congenital idiopathic clubfeet that fail to respond to nonoperative treatment, recurrent deformity after previous unsuccessful soft-tissue surgery, feet that show increasing deformity after apparent correction with prior nonoperative or operative treatment.

Surgical Age.   The optimum age for surgery is considered to be between 1 and 2 years of age. (Reasons will be discussed later.) In the initial reports on this operation the recommended upper age limit was 6 years. Subsequent experience has shown that in selected cases the age limit can be extended to 8 years. In the older age group, the alternative to soft-tissue surgery is a triple arthrodesis at skeletal maturity.

When it is suspected or evident that the deformity is due to a myopathy, neurologic deficit, or a genetic syndrome, early surgery should be avoided. In these cases it is recommended that surgery be delayed and carried out only when the deformity is such that surgical correction is mandatory after nonoperative methods fail to maintain a plantigrade foot. Surgery should also be postponed in cases that have considerably more than the usual plantar flexion of the talus, with some of the earmarks of a plantar flexed talus.

Technique.   A posterior medial plantar and subtalar release of all soft-tissue contractures is carried out in a one-stage operation. After the contractures are released, the navicular and calcaneus are restored to their normal relationship with the talus, and the surgical correction is stablized by temporarily transfixing the talonavicular and talocalcaneal joints with percutaneous Kirschner (K-) wires. In the older children a Steindler plantar stripping is also done when required. It is necessary to emphasize again that soft tissue contractures will vary in each case, even in bilateral deformities; the findings between the two sides vary. In each case, one must transect all soft-tissue contractures that prevent mobilization of the navicular and calcaneus in order to restore normal tarsal relationships.

The following discussion includes the abnormal anatomy that has been noted in the surgical correction of many and varied deformities. As with all operative procedures, attention to the details will avoid complications and insure an optimum result for each deformity confronting the surgeon.

Skin incision (Fig. 7-1A). A pneumatic tourniquet is used. The child is placed in the supine position with a sandbag or folded towel under the buttocks of the opposite side. The skin incision is made along the medial border of the foot. Beginning at the proximal end of the first metatarsal, the incision is extended proximally to just below the medial malleolus and continued posteriorly to the tendoachilles. In the older patient, and in patient's who have had prior surgery, it is advantageous to extend the incision slightly along the course of the achilles tendon; excessive vertical extension of the incision is not necessary. The tip of the medial malleolus is usually underdeveloped and difficult to palpate especially in chubby feet. In these cases, it helps to use a skin marker over the landmarks.

Exposure (Fig. 7-1B). The operation is essentially an anatomic dissection of the medial, plantar, and posterior aspects of the foot and ankle. Adequate surgical exposure is necessary to perform a meticulous dissection under direct vision to avoid traumatizing articular surfaces of the tarsal anlagen. Because of the tarsal displacement and the extensive fibrosis, dissection in a small deformed foot is difficult. The operation is facilitated by identifying and exposing the following five structures: posterior tibial tendon, flexor digitorum longus, posterior neurovascular bundle, flexor hallucis longus, and achilles tendon. As the tendons are exposed, the contracted tendon sheaths are incised thereby eliminating these contractures, which also contribute to the resistance.

The posterior tibial tendon is exposed by making a linear incision just below the medial malleolus, taking care not to incise the bone. Lysis of the tendon sheath is carried out from its insertion proximally above the ankle. In a clubfoot, the tendon is more vertically oriented than in the normal foot. Above the malleolus, the tendon appears cylindrical, while between the malleolus and the navicular, the tendon looses its cylindrical shape and appears as a broad expansion that blends with a mass of indistinguishable scar in this area.

The flexor digitorum longus is identified by making another linear incision just below the posterior tibial tendon. Because of the scar tissue, the flexor digitorum longus may be mistaken for the posterior tibial tendon, but are readily distinguished from each other by exerting traction on the exposed tendon.

The neurovascular bundle is located just below the long toe flexor. It is readily identified by the bluish discoloration of the posterior tibial vein. The nerve, artery, and vein are carefully exposed in their common sheath by blunt dissection and the bundle is retracted with a rubber, tissue Penrose drain. It is essential that the bundle be mobilized proximally and distally, so that all of the pathologic contractures can be transected under direct vision by retracting the bundle anteriorly or posteriorly during the dissection. The bundle must be mobilized distally under the abductor hallucis to the point where the posterior tibial nerve divides into its medial and lateral branches, when possible the calcaneal branch is preserved.

The flexor hallucis longus is identified by retracting the neurovascular bundle. In cases with extensive fibrosis, especially after prior surgery, passive flexion and

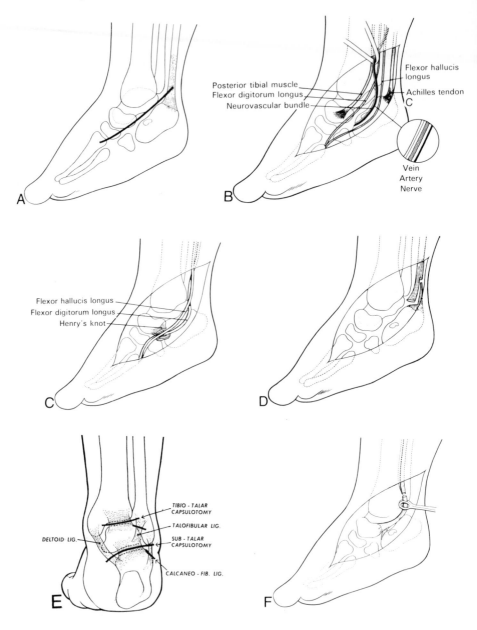

Fig. 7-1. *(A)* Skin Incision. *(B)* Anatomical exposure. *(C)* Master knot of Henry. *(D)* "Z" lengthening of tendo-Achilles. *(E)* Posterior capsulotomies of ankle and subtalar joints. Transection of posterior talofibular and calcaneofibular ligaments. *(F)* Posterior tibial tendon transection. The tendon may be lengthened by cutting all its plantar attachments, leaving only its insertion on the navicular tuberosity. (Turco, V. J.: Surgical correction of the resistant clubfoot. One-stage posteromedial release with internal fixation: A preliminary report. Journal of Bone and Joint Surgery, *53A:*477, 1971.)

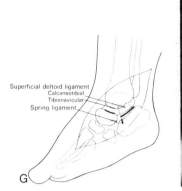

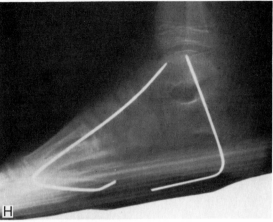

Superficial deltoid ligament
Calcaneotibial
Tibionavicular
Spring ligament

G

H

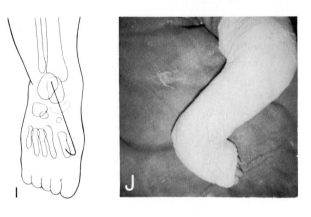

I

J

Fig. 7-1 *(continued)*. *(G)* Medial-plantar release. *(H)* K-wire transfixion of talocalcaneal joint. *(I)* K-wire transfixion of talonavicular joint. *(J)* Post operative cast.

extension of the big toe will help locate the tendon proximal to the mass of scar tissue.

The Achilles tendon is exposed after the neurovascular bundle is retracted anteriorly. The distal 2 to 3 cm of the Achilles tendon is exposed, including the broad insertion on the posterior tuberosity of the calcaneus.

The medial plantar dissection is completed by transecting the *master knot of Henry* (Fig. 7-1C). This fibrocartilagenous structure, which is attached to the undersurface of the navicular envelops the flexor digitorum longus and the flexor hallucis longus where they cross. It can be considered a localized hypertrophy of their tendon sheaths. Excision of the master knot is necessary to completely mobilize the navicular and permit transection of the spring ligament. The neurovascular bundle is retracted plantard, as the master knot is transected by continuing the lysis of the flexor tendon sheaths distally under the navicular. The technique is similiar to doing a lysis for a stenosing tenosynovitis of the flexor tendons in the hand. This plantar dissection also serves to detach abnormal attachments of the abductor hallucis from the posterior tibial tendon, navicular tuberosity, and the first metatarsal, when this abnormal origin is present. Some of the contractures are eliminated with this surgical exposure. After this part of the operation is completed, it is well to assess the abnormal tarsal relationship before correction; notice that the posterior tuberosity of the calcaneus is pulled upward; the navicular and sustentaculum tali are displaced medially closer to the malleolus; and on passive dorsiflexion and plantar flexion the excursion of the posterior end of the calcaneus is limited and the navicular is immobile. After the five structures have been identified and mobilized, incision of the remaining pathologic contractures is performed in three steps: the posterior release, the medial plantar release, and the subtalar release.

Posterior Release. *(Tendo Achilles lengthening (TAL), capsulotomy of tibiotalar joint, capsulotomy talocalcaneal joint, transection posterior talofibular ligament, transection calcaneofibular ligament)*

Experience with the operation has shown that doing the posterior release first facilitates exposure and excision of the medial plantar and the subtalar contractures. In the clubfoot, the Achilles insertion on the calcaneus is broader and more distal and medial than in the normal foot. For this reason, the tendon is lengthened by the "Z" technique in the sagittal plane, detaching the medial one-half of the insertion on the calcaneus and thereby eliminating the inversion force of the tendo achillis. Excessive lengthening is unnecessary. One should plan to lengthen the tendon just enough to permit immobilization at an angle of approximately 90° (Fig. 7-1*D*). Anterior retraction of the neurovascular bundle and the flexor hallucis longus brings into view the posterior aspect of the ankle joint. A capsulotomy of the ankle joint is done before the capsulotomy of the subtalar joint (Fig. 7-1*E*); if the talocalcaneal capsulotomy is done first, identification and the capsulotomy of the ankle joint are more difficult.

The posterior capsulotomy is more difficult in patients who have had previous surgery; even a simple Achilles lengthening or percutaneous lengthening of Achilles will cause scarring in this area. The most extensive and dense scarring has been noted when in the previous surgery, a K-wire had been inserted in the calcaneus and incorporated in the cast to pull the posterior tuberosity downward. The ankle joint is also quite difficult to identify when there is marked plantar flexion of the talus. In these feet, the visible posterior trochlea of the talus is wafer thin and care must be taken to avoid iatrogenic injury to the bone and joint surfaces. Passive upward and downward movement of the ankle joint helps to locate the tibiotalar joint. After the ankle joint is identified, first a small opening is made in the capsule and then the capsulotomy is completed under direct vision by cutting from within out. When the posterior talofibular ligament is also contracted, it can be transected by extending the capsulotomy laterally to the fibular side. A common error is to extend the capsulotomy of the ankle too far forward, thereby transecting the deep deltoid attachment on the medial surface of the talus. The deep deltoid must be preserved medially to avoid "talar tilt" out of the mortise. Next, the posterior talocalcaneal joint is identified and transected with the calcaneofibular ligament, as in the tibiotalar joint. The lateral ligaments of the ankle are more commonly found contracted in older children. In some cases, one may find minimal fibrosis of the tibiotalar joint capsule; however, invariably the talocalcaneal capsule is contracted.

The final step in the posterior release is to incise the posterior portion of the deltoid attachment on the calcaneus. This is readily accomplished by extending the capsulotomy of the posterior subtalar joint slightly forward. After the subtalar joint has been identified medially, attention is then directed to elimination of the medial plantar contractures. At this point in the operation, it is well to assess how much correction has been attained by the posterior release alone. This is done by dorsiflexing the foot and reexamining the relationship of the navicular and sustentaculum tali to the medial malleolus. Evaluation reveals that the posterior release alone corrects very little of the equinus deformity; the calcaneus is still locked in varus under the talus and the navicular is still rigidly fixed in its medially displaced position.

Medial Plantar Release. *(Posterior tibial tendon, superficial deltoid ligament, talonavicular capsule, spring ligament)*

The flexor digitorum longus and flexor hallucis longus are retracted together in a Penrose drain or tape. Retraction of the flexor tendons dorsally and the neurovascular bundle plantard brings into view a mass of indistinguishable fibrous tissue composed of the broad attachments of the posterior tibial tendon, deltoid ligament, talonavicular capsule, and spring ligament. This mass of scar tissue, plus the medially displaced navicular, obscures the midtarsal and subtalar joints as well as the neck of the talus. This mass of contractures must be transected in order to mobilize the navicular and the anterior end of the calcaneus. Dissection of this mass of cicatrix is the most important and difficult part of the operation and must be done without damaging bones and joint surfaces. Complete mobilization of the navicular and the anterior end of the calcaneus is essential for a successful operation. Failure to completely release the contractures in this area is one of the technical errors responsible for surgical failure. The author has noted, during surgery following failures of prior one-stage PMR, that this region is often surgically virgin.

Mobilization of the navicular is begun by cutting the posterior tibial tendon at the level of the malleolus (Fig. 7-1*F*). If the surgeon prefers to lengthen the posterior tibial tendon, it is imperative to cut all of its broad accessory attachments, leaving only the insertion on the navicular tuberosity intact. Traction on the distal stump of the posterior tibial tendon facilitates transection of the deltoid attachment on the navicular and the talonavicular capsule. This technique also precludes the danger of damaging joint surfaces. After the initial incision is made in the talonavicular capsule, the glistening head of the talus is seen deep in the wound, and the anterior tibial tendon is retracted laterally, thereby protecting the dorsalis pedis artery while the talonavicular capsulotomy is completed dorsomedially. While mobilizing the navicular, one should keep in mind that the talonavicular joint faces medially in a more sagittal plane, rather than in the normal coronal orientation. The posterior tibial attachments to the sustentaculum tali and the spring ligament are incised. The plantar release is completed by incising the spring ligament anterior to the sustentaculum tali and under the head of the talus (Fig. 7-1*G*).

The medial release is then completed by returning to the site of the posterior release that ended with the identification of the subtalar joint. The calcaneus is everted as the capsulotomy of the subtalar joint is extended forward (Fig. 7-1*G*). Transection of this contracture is done by inserting a snap in the subtalar joint, then opening the snap to distract the calcaneus, thereby permitting excision of the contracture by cutting from within outward. The degree of displacement and the size of the sustentaculum tali vary. In the region of the sustentaculum tali, invariably one finds a dense mass of fibrocartilagenous scar tissue interposed between the sustentaculum tali, the navicular, and the malleolus. This scar binds the sustentaculum and navicular medially to the talus and closer to the medial malleolus; the joint margins are completely obscured by this scar. Excision of this scar tissue is best done by a combination of blunt and cautious sharp dissection to avoid excision of the sustentaculum tali. The mass of scar is probed a little at a time with the point of a snap as the snap is opened to spread the contractures, which are then cut by cautious sharp dissection between the open ends of the snap, under direct vision. All of this contracture must be released in order to mobilize the navicular and the anterior end of the calcaneus. The deep deltoid attachment on the talus is preserved.

Subtalar Release.   *(Talocalcaneo interosseous ligament; bifurcated Y-ligament)*

The subtalar release completes the mobilization of the calcaneus and navicular. In children, 1 year old or younger the talocalcaneal ligament is usually less contracted than in the older patient. Release of the interosseous ligament should be limited to the amount necessary to unlock the calcaneus to allow eversion and abduction. Complete transection of the interosseous ligament can produce a severe valgus deformity and should be avoided. Usually it is necessary to transect only the medial portion of the ligament.

The interosseous ligament is exposed by everting the heel manually and it is cut under direct vision. When the contractures of the subtalar joint are extremely rigid and hypertrophied, it may be necessary to insert a snap in the subtalar joint to distract the calcaneus by opening the snap. When the interosseous ligament is extremely dense and thickened, forceful eversion of the heel before the interosseous ligament is released should be avoided. Excessive valgus force can produce an avulsion fracture as the intact ligament pulls away an osteochondral fragment from the top of the calcaneus. Less commonly, the Y-ligament may prevent complete mobilization of the navicular and the anterior end of the calcaneus. This contracture is located distal to the interosseous ligament and can be easily transected, if necessary, through the medial approach.

Navicular-cuneiform capsulotomy is done when there appears to be significant medial displacement of the cuneiform on the navicular. The capsulotomy of this joint is limited to the medial aspect in order to minimize impairment of the blood supply to the navicular.

Internal Fixation

The surgical correction is stablized by transfixing the talocalcaneal and talonavicular joints with percutaneous Kirschner wires (0.45 mm). In the original technique, only the talonavicular joint was transfixed. When only the talonavicular joint is stabilized, the correction is maintained. However, the heel can evert because the foot may rotate around the horizontal pin when the foot is placed in dorsiflexion in the postoperative care. To prevent this, the subtalar joint is also stabilized. Excessive valgus angulation of the heel must be avoided. While overcorrection is very difficult with closed treatment, it can be easily accomplished after this extensive soft-tissue release.

The subtalar joint is transfixed first by a vertical percutaneous Kirschner wire that is introduced from below into the body of the talus while the calcaneus is held in the desired corrected position. The ankle joint is not included. The heel pad should be displaced medially before the wire is inserted in order to avoid transfixing the skin laterally, thereby making wound closure difficult (Fig. 7-1*H*).

Care must be taken not to overcorrect the navicular laterally on the head of the talus. This will produce a severe pes planus; one must also avoid placing the navicular too far dorsad. In feet with a fairly normal talar head, it is easier to decide the optimum position for the navicular. When the head of the talus is quite deformed, it is very difficult to decide the optimum position of the navicular. In this situation, it is best to estimate the relationship of the head and neck to the body, paying particular attention to the degree of equinus, then "eye ball" the placement of the navicular.

While the navicular is held in the corrected position, the horizontal K-wire is inserted percutaneously from the dorsum of the foot across the talonavicular joint into the head, neck, and body of the talus (Fig. 7.1*H*). Some surgeons have reported modifications of this technique by inserting the Kirschner wire retrograde through the articular surface of the navicular; others have inserted the wire retrograde through the posterior aspect of the trochlea. For the insertion of both the talocalcaneal and talonavicular wires, it is important that the surgeon observe the wires penetrating the joints in the desired position to make certain the bones are rigidly transfixed. Overlooking this little detail can result in a technical failure with loss of correction. The depth of penetration into the talus is measured by placing a wire of similiar length adjacent to the wire inserted into the foot. A power drill has facilitated the insertion of K-wires.

After both wires are inserted, the relationship of the calcaneus and the navicular on the talus must be carefully inspected to make certain the bones are in the desired position, the correction is stable, and the ankle joint is mobile. The protruding wires are bent, then cut, leaving 2 to 3 cm of the bent wire. It is recommended that the wires be cut in this manner, with the long ends protruding in order to prevent the wires from falling out. This complication has been reported, by colleagues, as a cause of technical error and loss of correction. The cast is more effective in preventing an outward migration on a long piece of bent wire, compared to a short end that is more likely to be extruded, especially in the initially well-padded postoperative cast of an active child. The K-wires should not be incorporated in the plaster cast because invariably they will fall out, also this technique complicates the initial cast change.

Achilles Repair—Postoperative Immobilization

In the past, excessive heel-cord lengthening was a recommended and common practice. Excessive TAL is unnecessary; it serves only to increase the calf atrophy and weakness common to all clubfeet. Excessive lengthening and calf atrophy are minimized with the following technique of repairing the "Z" plasty of the achilles: before suturing the tendon, the proximal end is pulled distally to "take up all the slack," and the two ends are sutured side to side while the foot is held at a right angle, without any "slack" of the distal segment. If the posterior tibial tendon is lengthened, the anastomosis is preferably performed above the malleolus to avoid scarring over the midtarsal and subtalar joints.

Before closure of the wound, the foot is gently forced into dorsiflexion to evaluate the maximum dorsiflexion possible after the release. Full dorsiflexion is usually limited by impingement of the overgrown anterior trochlea and the neck of the talus; this is more pronounced in the older child and in cases with severe preoperative equinus. When there is marked limitation of dorsiflexion due to this overgrowth, the range of dorsiflexion is gradually increased postoperatively with more frequent cast changes to allow the talus to remold gradually as more of the trochlea enters the ankle joint. In this situation, one must also consider leaving the K-wires in place longer to prevent increasing heel valgus or dorsal subluxation of the navicular, which are more apt to occur in these cases during postoperative manipulation after the K-wires are removed. The subcutaneous tissues are closed with fine absorbable sutures; synthetic absorbable sutures for skin closure has eliminated the hassle of suture removal in children. A small piece of felt is placed between the bent wire and the skin and a separate piece of gauze dressing is applied over each wire under the sheet wadding to avoid the danger of pulling the wire out with the cast padding during cast removal. A well-padded above-knee case is applied with the knee in flexion (Fig. 71J). The degree of initial dorsiflexion is determined by the severity of the skin contracture and impingement of the talus on the anterior lip of the tibia. Usually the foot is immobilized at about a right angle to avoid tension necrosis of the contracted skin. In the corrected position, a plantar flexion of the big toe, and occasionally the lesser toes, is usually observed. This is a normal occurrence and results from lengthening of the preoperative medial concavity of the foot. The shortened tendons elongate without sequelae.

POSTOPERATIVE CARE—INFANCY

All feet are different. Therefore, identical routine postoperative care is not applicable in all cases. However, postoperative treatment is as important as the surgery, and sucess requires that management after surgical correction be tailored for each case, depending on the findings, and the age of the patient. The following should serve as a guide to postoperative care.

Guide to Postoperative Management. Three weeks after surgery, the cast is changed under general anesthesia. In removing the cast, care is taken to prevent the K-wires from falling out. After skin care, a new above-knee cast is applied, with the foot in more dorsiflexion. At 6 weeks, the cast is changed in the office. Initially, it had been recommended that internal fixation be removed at 6 weeks; this practice has been modified as follows: The K-wires are removed at 6 weeks if full dorsiflexion is possible and there is no danger of causing severe heel valgus or dorsal subluxation of the navicular as the foot is dorsiflexed; the K-wires are removed at 6 weeks when full dorsiflexion is readily possible at this time and if the evaluation of the range of dorsiflexion at the time of surgery showed no evidence of marked impingement of the talus on the anterior lip of the tibia. It is recommended that the wires be left in place for several weeks longer in the following situations: when dorsiflexion is limited because the talus impinges on the anterior lip of the tibia; the talus is markedly plantar flexed because these feet are predisposed to develop planovalgus; there is a danger of dorsal subluxation of the navicular as the foot is dorsiflexed (Fig. 7-2), in the case of chubby feet and fat legs and

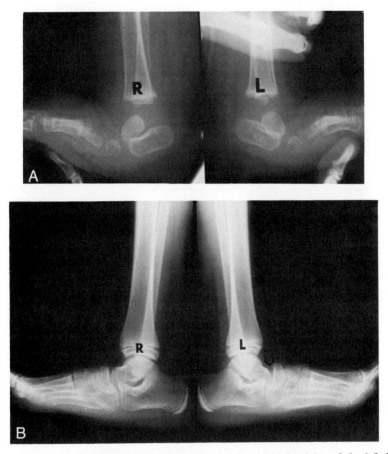

Fig. 7-2. This case illustrates dorsal subluxation of the navicular joint of the left foot of a 12-year-old child. The child had bilateral rocker-bottom deformities. One-stage PMR with internal fixation was done at age 1 year, and internal fixation was removed 6 weeks after surgery. Dorsal displacement of the navicular joint occurred when dorsiflexion was increased after removal of the internal fixation. This occurrence can be avoided by continuing the internal fixation several weeks longer than usual in cases such as this. Dorsal subluxation is more apt to occur when the talus is markedly plantar flexed, as in rocker-bottom, and when dorsiflexion is restricted by impingment of the anterior trochlea on the anterior lip of the tibia. This abnormal talonavicular relationship can also be the result of transfixing the navicular joint in a dorsal position on a broad, deformed head of the talus. *(A)* Bilateral rocker-bottom deformity. *(B)* Radiographs showing weight bearing at age 13. Note the dorsal subluxation of the navicular on the left side.

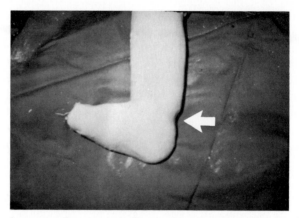

Fig. 7-3.   Above-knee cast after removal of internal fixation. Note that the plaster is molded above the posterior tuberosity of the heel to insure that the cast maintains the surgical correction.

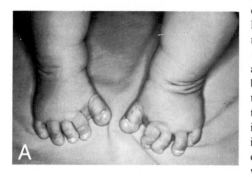

Fig. 7-4   Illustrative case. This case is an example of postoperative cast slippage with loss of surgical correction in plaster after removal of the internal fixation. The child *(A)* aged 16 months, has short, stubby feet and fat legs and thighs; because of this his bilateral resistant feet are especially difficult to maintain in corrective casts. Preoperative radiographs of the left foot are shown in *(B)*. Bilateral posteromedial release with internal fixation was done at 16 months of age. At 6 weeks after surgery the "K" wires were removed and correction was complete.

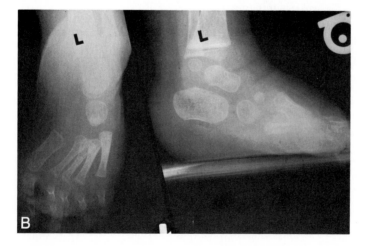

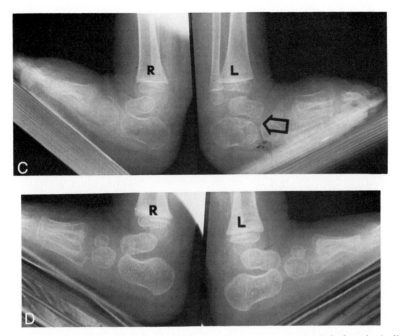

Fig. 7-4 *(continued)*. By 10 weeks postoperatively, the cast on the left foot had slipped. Radiographs showed that the correction on the left side was lost *(C)*. Note on the left foot the calcaneus and talus are parallel, the sinus tarsi is open, and there is no dorsiflexion of the heel. The left foot appears similiar to the preoperative radiographs. Correction on the right side is satisfactory. A course of weekly serial manipulations and above-knee corrective casts was continued until full correction was regained. Radiographs 6 months after surgery confirmed the clinical evaluation of a good correction bilaterally *(D)*. A corrective plaster splint was used at night and naptime for an additional 4 months and then replaced with a D-B bar with attached corrective shoes.

thighs, which are very difficult to retain corrected in plaster after internal fixation is removed; and in talocalcaneal synchondrosis. There have been no ill effects from leaving K-wires in place longer than 6 weeks. While the K-wires are in the foot, the cast should extend above the knee to discourage the child from walking with internal fixation. In children under 3 years of age, a long leg cast with the knee flexed to 90° is now used routinely after internal fixation is removed to insure that the correction is maintained.

Although internal fixation maintains surgical correction; it can be lost in plaster after the wires are removed, especially in children with "baby fat." Loss of correction after wire removal is prevented by applying a snug-fitting cast similar to that used for initial manipulation and cast treatment. One layer of cast padding is used, and the plaster must be well-molded above the posterior tuberosity to lock the heel in the corrected position (Fig. 7-3). The child's parents are warned to keep checking the protrusion of the toes out of the cast; toe retraction is evidence of cast slippage and failure to maintain correction. When slippage is detected, a good result can be obtained and recurrent deformity prevented by corrective manip-

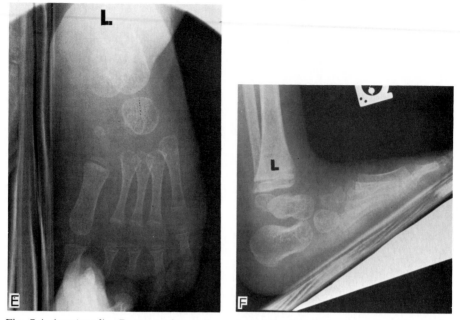

Fig. 7-4 *(continued).* Postoperative radiographs of the left foot taken after 10 months *(E)* and 2 years *(F)* show that a lasting correction was salvaged. This was possible because of early detection of loss of surgical correction due to cast slippage and because serial corrective manipulations were instituted for a period longer than the usual postoperative plaster immobilization. In cases such as this, it is recommended that the internal fixation be continued a few weeks longer than usual and that extra care taken to apply a snug, long-leg cast with careful observation for evidence of cast slippage.

ulations and serial casts beyond the usual 4 months of postoperative plaster immobilization. The author has had six cases of cast slippage, which were detected in time and went on to successful results following serial manipulations and cast treatment (Fig. 7-4).

After the K-wires are removed, the plaster casts are changed as often as is necessary for a total of 4 months. The last cast is a below-knee walking cast to provide a physiologic stimulus for remolding the articular surfaces while the foot is being held in the corrected position (Fig. 7-5). After 4 months of immobilization in plaster, the child uses a Denis Browne (D-B) Bar (25 cm), with attached open-toe corrective shoes, during sleeping hours for a minimum of 1 year (Fig. 7-6); straight last shoes are used for walking. Illustrative cases are shown in Figs. 7-7 and 7-8.

Case 1 (Fig. 7-7), shows a right clubfoot that was treated from birth with serial manipulations and casts. At 7 months of age, dorsiflexion was equal to the right. The correction was maintained in a D-B Bar. Several months later the mother noted increasing tightness of the heel cord and difficulty applying and maintaining the right foot in the shoe. At 14 months a one-stage PMR with internal fixation was done. The preoperative radiographs showed apparent correction with good

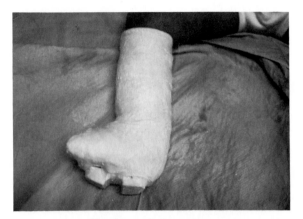

Fig. 7-5.   Walking Cast.

divergence of the hindfoot in the antero-posterior view (Fig. 7-7*A*). However the lateral view showed no dorsiflexion of the calcaneus (Fig. 7-7*B*). At 16 years of age, the right foot was cosmetically acceptable and pliable (Fig. 7-7*C*). The young-ster played all sports and had a normal gait but slight calf atrophy. The radiographs at skeletal maturity confirmed that the correction had been maintained (Fig. 7-7*D*, *E*).

Illustrative Case 2 (Fig. 7-8) shows a 4-year-old boy who was initially seen with a large, painful callous and severe recurrent deformity after two previous operations. A posterior release was done at one year, a medial release at 2 years

(continued on page 131)

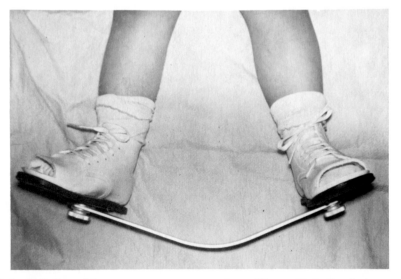

Fig. 7-6.   D-B Bar with open-toe tarsopronator shoes. (Turco, V. J.: Surgical correction of the resistant clubfoot. One-stage posteromedial release with internal fixation: A preliminary report. Journal of Bone and Joint Surgery, *53A:*477, 1971.)

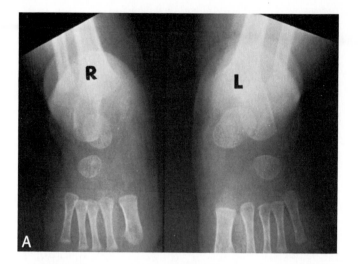

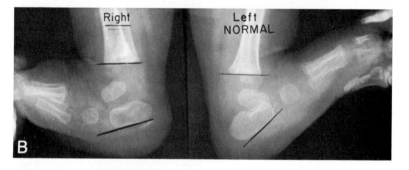

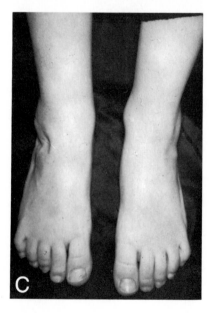

Fig. 7-7.   *(A)* Right clubfoot at 14 months. Radiographs show apparent divergence of the hindfoot. Note tarsal bones are smaller in the clubfoot. *(B)* Preoperative dorsiflexion lateral view shows no dorsiflexion of the calcaneus on the right. *(C)* Weight-bearing photograph at 16 years. (*B* from Turco, V. J.: Surgical correction of the resistant clubfoot. One-stage posteromedial release with internal fixation: A preliminary report. Journal of Bone and Joint Surgery, *53A:*477, 1971.)

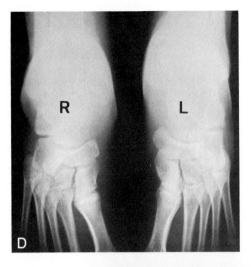

Fig. 7-7 *(continued).* *(D)* Radiographs at skeletal maturity show normal tarsal relationship in comparison with the normal left foot. *(E)* Dorsiflexion at 16 years is equal. Note the slight residual abnormality of the talus in the right clubfoot.

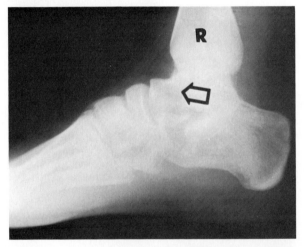

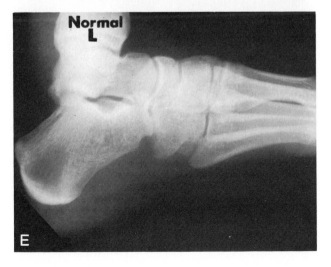

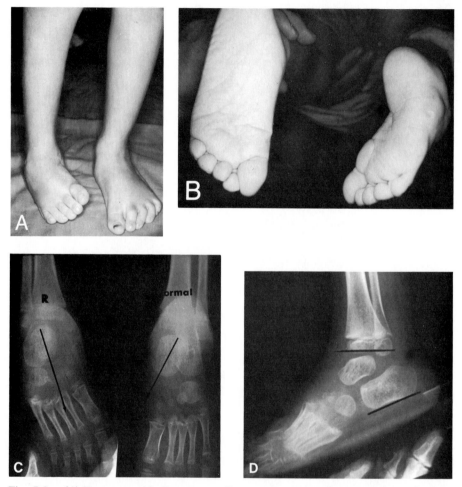

Fig. 7-8. *(A)* Four-year old. Recurrent talipes equinovarus, after two prior soft tissue operations. *(B)* Painful callous over dorsal aspect of 5th right metatarsal, with bean-shaped deformity. *(C)* Preoperative radiograph with comparison view. *(D)* Dorsiflexion lateral view shows limited dorsiflexion of the calcaneus. Note deformity in the trochlea and neck of the talus.

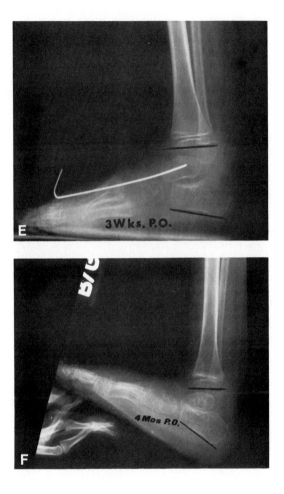

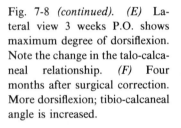

Fig. 7-8 *(continued)*. *(E)* Lateral view 3 weeks P.O. shows maximum degree of dorsiflexion. Note the change in the talo-calcaneal relationship. *(F)* Four months after surgical correction. More dorsiflexion; tibio-calcaneal angle is increased.

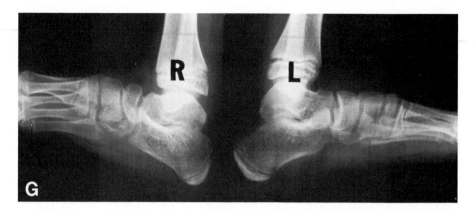

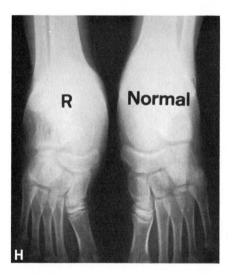

Fig. 7-8 *(continued).* *(G)* Lateral dorsiflexion at 13 years. Full dorsiflexion of right clubfoot. Remolding of the talus make it possible for all of the trochlea to enter the mortise. *(H)* Thirteen years of age. Normal tarsal relationship. *(I)* Plantar view. No callosities, bean-shaped deformity of right clubfoot corrected. *(J)* Weight Bearing.

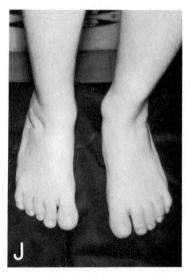

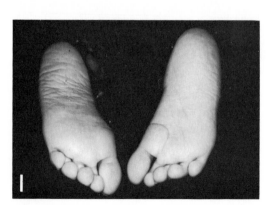

of age. The mother noted that the deformity was increasing and the child was having difficulty running. A one-stage PMR was done at 4 years. Preoperatively there was significant equinovarus deformity. (Figs. 7-8*A, B*). Radiographs showed an uncorrected deformity (Figs. 7-8*C, D*). Reduction of the navicular was impossible until the bifurcated "Y" ligament was transected. The contracted skin and deformity of the talus limited dorsiflexion to a right angle after surgical correction (Fig. 8-8*E*). In the postoperative management, the casts were changed at 3-week intervals as dorsiflexion was gradually increased at each manipulation. The internal fixation was removed 9 weeks postoperatively. By 4 months after surgery, full dorsiflexion was possible (Fig. 7-8*F*). Correction was maintained in a corrective plaster splint at night for one year. The radiographs showed normal tarsal relationship and full dorsiflexion (Fig. 7-8*G, H*). At 13 years, the foot was plantigrade, pliable. The youngster participated normally in all activities (Fig. 7-8*I, J*).

Technique in Patients with Severe Cavus Deformity

In the younger children, a severe cavus component is usually associated with a deep cleft in the plantar surface of the foot. In the older child, over 5 years old, the plantar aponeurosis is contracted without a deep cleft in the plantar surface of the foot. When cavus deformity is present, the roentgenograms show a plantar-flexed first metatarsal. At operation, one usually finds the anterior tibial tendon inserting more distally on the shaft of the first metatarsal and an abnormal, more dorsal, origin of the abductor hallucis with attachments on the posterior tibial tendon sheath and the navicular tuberosity. The abnormal anterior tibial attachment on the first metatarsal is deleted, leaving only the proximal normal insertion intact. I have not transplanted the anterior tibial tendon laterally in these feet. Rather than section the insertion of the abductor hallucis, it is preferable to detach its abnormal origin. This is accomplished during the surgical exposure when the posterior tibial tendon and the two flexor tendons are lysed from their contracted sheaths. With this technique, the abductor hallucis is readily released from its abnormal accessory origin.

In older children with severe cavus, a Steindler[36] plantar stripping is done at the same operation, before the one-stage release. A separate longitudinal incision 2 to 3 cm long is made over the contracted plantar fasica along the medial plantar surface, just distal to the heel (Fig. 7-9*A*). Through this incision, the plantar fascia is cut. Then the origin of the abductor hallucis and the intrinsic toe flexors are stripped subperiosteally from the plantar surface of the calcaneus. (This is the only time a periosteal elevator is used in soft-tissue clubfoot surgery.) This incision is located lateral and proximal to the posterior tibial nerve, and there have been no problems with this incision on the medial plantar surface of the foot (Fig. 7-9*B*). When a Steindler stripping is done, the incision for the one-stage release is made slightly more dorsad. In the older child, the overgrown tuberosity of the navicular may be quite prominent after reduction, may be excised to prevent pressure on the skin.

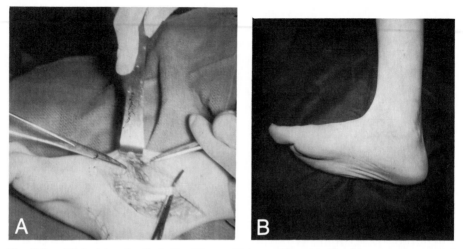

Fig. 7-9.   *(A)* Incision for Steindler Plantar Release. Six-year-old with severe cavus and equinovarus deformities. The Steindler stripping is done first through this medial-plantar incision. *(B)* At 15 years. Active dorsiflexion. The plantar incision is hardly visible.

Intraoperative Assessment of the Correction

After the posteromedial plantar and subtalar release have been completed, the deformity can be corrected without force. Surgical correction is assessed to make certain it is complete and all contractures have been cut in the following manner: first the foot is placed in the position of initial deformity and the relationship of the navicular and calcaneus to the talus are noted; attention then is focused on the movement and the final corrected position of the navicular, sustentaculum tali, and the posterior tuberosity of the calcaneus. Notice that as the foot is placed in the corrected position the navicular and the calcaneus move together as the foot rotates laterally around the talus. In the corrected foot, the navicular moves forward and anterior to the head of the talus, the anterior end of the calcaneus moves laterally as the sustentaculum assumes a more normal position under the talus, and the subtalar joint opens like a book, as the posterior tuberosity of the calcaneus moves downward. Notice that all three components of the deformity are corrected simultaneously. After the bony deformity is corrected, there is an empty space between the medial adjacent surfaces of the talus and the calcaneus. This open-book appearance is to be expected with eversion of the previously inverted calcaneus. The empty space is exaggerated because of underdevelopment of the adjacent surfaces of the calcaneus and talus, secondary to the persistent medial compression in the fixed varus position. Initially, this void along the medial subtalar joint was a source of concern, but experience has shown that after correction, remolding takes place.

Postoperative Management—Older Child.   Postoperative care for the older child is slightly different for these reasons: there is more deformity of the anterior trochlea and neck thus a greater factor in limiting dorsiflexion; remolding takes longer; it is easier to apply an effective cast; the D-B bar cannot be used in this age group; and the older child is prone to develop flatfeet. As for the infant, the initial cast is changed at 3 weeks under anesthesia, and a second, above-knee plaster cast is applied with the foot held in more dorsiflexion. The casts are changed more frequently, and on each change of cast dorsiflexion is increased. The wires are removed at 8 weeks, but if necessary they may be left in place longer. Walking casts are applied when maintenance of correction is assured. After 4 to 5 months of plaster immobilization, a bivalved plaster cast is used to maintain the correction at night. The child and parents are instructed in peroneal strengthening exercises, and the child is also instructed to walk alternately on their heels and toes in order to strengthen dorsiflexors as well as the triceps.

Advantages of One-Stage PMR

The most important advantage of the one-stage procedure is that a complete correction is attained when equinus, varus, and adduction deformities are eliminated in the same operation. It is impossible to completely correct any one component without correcting the others. The calcaneus is involved in all three components of deformity: equinus, varus, and adduction. It is not possible to correct the equinus of the heel completely without also eliminating the varus adduction components of the deformity; the opposite is also true. For dorsiflexion, the posterior tuberosity of the calcaneus must be free to move downward while the anterior end must also be mobilized to evert and move laterally around the talus. At the same time, the navicular moves laterally with the anterior end of the calcaneus. One-stage PMR mobilizes both ends of the calcaneus and the navicular to permit restoration of the normal anatomy and mechanics necessary for dorsiflexion. In the past, the author utilized the two-stage medial-posterior release and also a posterior release alone. These techniques produced unsatisfactory results, except in mild deformities, because these piecemeal operations attained incomplete corrections. The posterior release alone decreases the equinus deformity of the ankle; it does not change the equinus and varus deformity of the calcaneus. After a posterior release, the relationship between the calcaneus and talus remains the same because the calcaneus is still locked in varus under the talus. This is the reason for the high incidence of recurrent deformities after posterior release alone. When only the medial release is done in a severe deformity, very little of the varus is correctable, because it is impossible to completely correct the deformity of the calcaneus while its posterior tuberosity is pulled upward by the posterior contractures. The correction of the abnormal position of the calcaneus can be compared to a log of wood bobbing up and down in waves at sea (Fig. 7-10). As one end of the log moves downward (posterior tuberosity of calcaneus), the other end of the log (anterior end of oscalcis) moves in the opposite direction as it rolls on its side (eversion, abduction of calcaneus).

Advantages of Internal Fixation

Transfixion of the talonavicular and talocalcaneal joints insures maintenance of the surgical correction. The correction is maintained without cast pressure or

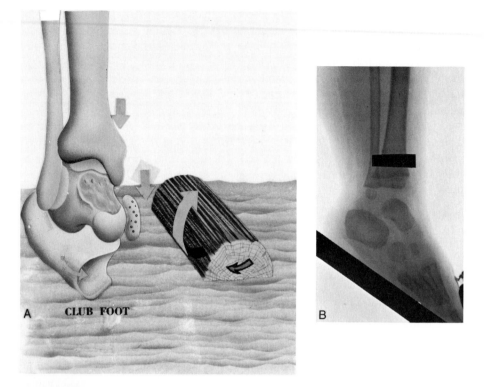

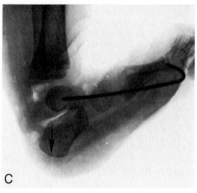

Fig. 7-10. *(A)* Correction of equinus, varus and adduction of the calcaneus is comparable to the movement of a log rolling in the sea. For the posterior tuberosity of the calcaneus to move downward, the anterior end must be free to move in the opposite direction as it rotates externally. *(B)* Preoperative radiograph of 2-year-old shows typical equinus deformity of calcaneus. *(C)* Intraoperative radiograph of same patient after one-state PMR. Note the posterior tuberosity has moved downward, the anterior end upward. The sinus tarsi is closed with correction of the fixed varus deformity.

hyperdorsiflexion of the foot, thus eliminating two causes of skin necrosis: pressure and tension on the wound. The cast serves as a protective splint rather than as a corrective device. Previously, when the same operation was done without internal fixation, there was a high incidence of problems with wound healing; the high incidence of recurrence deformity was attributable to failure to maintain the surgical correction in a plaster cast alone. In the long-term follow-up, no deleterious effects from the use of internal fixation have been noticed. By transfixing the talonavicular and subtalar joints, the relationship of the navicular, calcaneus, and talus remains constant as dorsiflexion is increased in postoperative care. Dorsal subluxation of the navicular and increased eversion of the calcaneus are prevented as more of the talus enters the mortise with increased dorsiflexion. Internal fixation is especially advantageous in the small child with severe equinovarus deformity, or in feet that have had previous operations. In these feet, the danger of skin necrosis is minimized by permitting initial immobilization in equinus (Fig. 7-11). This technique has an added advantage, in the older child, when overgrowth of the anterior trochlea and neck of the talus limits dorsiflexion. In these situations, when dorsiflexion is contraindicated or impossible, the initial immobilization may be in slight equinus, if necessary to prevent wound problems. The corrected relationship of the navicular, calcaneus, and talus is maintained while the three bones move en masse as more of the talus enters the ankle mortise with increased dorsiflexion postoperatively (Fig. 7-12).

Soft-Tissue Release in Older Children

Children older than 6 years, with a severe equinocavovarus deformity, present a difficult challenge. These children have usually been treated with braces after unsuccessful nonoperative and operative treatment. They present with a history of increasing deformity; their inability to get the foot into a shoe precludes their continued use of the brace. In the past, the recommendation for these cases was to have them "return at skeletal maturity for a triple arthrodesis."

The changes that develop in the shape of the trochlea and neck of the talus of an uncorrected foot at skeletal maturity point out the futility of doing nothing until that time. Secondary adaptive changes are superimposed on the initial deformity of the talus by the time the child reaches skeletal maturity, and the incongruity of the tibiotalar joint will preclude a good functional and cosmetic result with triple arthrodesis.

While the results of soft-tissue surgery in children more than 6 years of age are not as successful, they have been considered quite satisfactory, considering the severity of the deformity and age of the patient. Initially, the rationale for operating on this age group was to minimize the deformity to preserve the trochlea of the talus for a more successful, cosmetic and functional triple arthrodesis at maturity. The results in this group have been considered quite acceptable, since the alternative of triple arthrodesis was usually avoided. In the authors opinion, triple arthrodesis for a clubfoot is considered a salvage procedure and should be avoided, if possible. In patient's over the age of 6 years, a one-stage PMR should be done in selected cases. The prerequisites are a well-preserved trochlea, subtalar and midtarsal articular surfaces, and pliable skin that can withstand surgery. In this age group, soft-tissue surgery has demonstrated that the talus has a considerable capacity to remold in response to physiologic stress. These children usually require a Steindler plantar stripping in addition to the one-stage release. (Illustrative cases are shown in Figs. 7-13 and 7-14.) If there is any question regarding problems with healing of the surgical incision, the surgery should be staged. The Steindler plantar release is done first, and the one-stage PMR is done 3 to 4 weeks later.

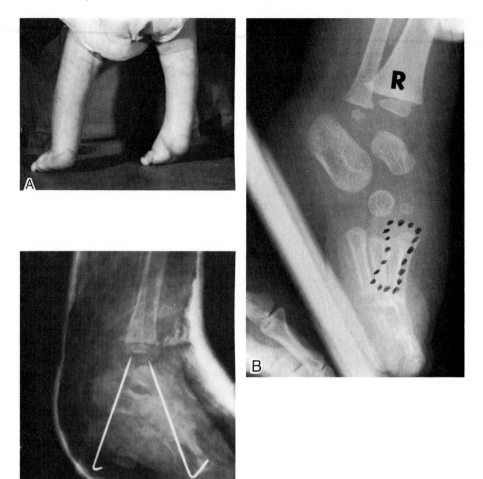

Fig. 7-11. This case illustrates the advantages of internal fixation in preventing complications of wound healing and heel valgus in a child with a severe equinocavus deformity associated with a severe degree of skin contracture. Bilateral one-stage PMR operations were done at 15 months. The contracted skin necessitated initial postoperative immobilization in equinus. A satisfactory result was obtained and skin complications were avoided by gradually increasing dorsiflexion after surgery. The internal fixation was removed 8 weeks postoperatively. *(A)* Age 15 months: bilateral deformity. Note the severe equinus, cavus and a deep plantar cleft of the right foot. *(B)* Preoperative lateral view with the foot held in maximum dorsiflexion. The talus appears to be subluxed anteriorly out of the mortise. At surgery, the body of the talus appeared wafer-thin in the posterior aspect of the ankle joint. Note the plantar-flexed first metatarsal, a common occurrence with severe cavus. The tibialis anterior tendon insertion extended down to the middle of the first metatarsal, the abductor hallucis had an acessory origin from the tendon sheath of the tibialis posterior and the navicular tuberosity. The abnormal origin and insertion of these structures were detached. *(C)* Postoperative radiograph shows the initial immobilization in equinus necessitated by the contracted skin.

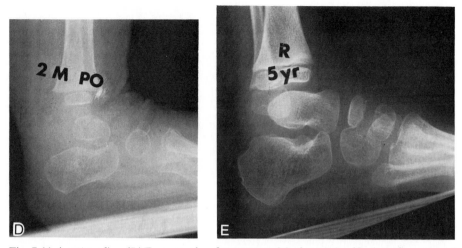

Fig. 7-11 *(continued).* *(D)* Two months after surgery. Maximum dorsiflexion after removal of internal fixation. *(E)* Age 5 years. Satisfactory result equinus cavus and varus corrected. Skin complications and heel valgus were avoided. (*A* from Journal of Bone and Joint Surgery, 61*A*, Sept. 1979.)

ONE-STAGE PMR WITH INTERNAL FIXATION— PERSONAL SERIES

This study is based on 16 years of experience with a one-stage PMR with internal fixation for resistant idiopathic clubfeet. The review includes results, complications, analyses of fair and poor results, and a report of unusual findings at the time of surgery.

Materials and Methods

The author was personally involved in the surgery of 273 feet with recalcitrant deformities that had failed to respond to nonoperative treatment or had previously been treated unsuccessfully by surgery. The feet were evaluated preoperatively and postoperatively, utilizing the same clinical and radiographic assessment. Many of the children in the series were treated from birth by the author, but most had received their initial treatment elsewhere and were seen for the first time after 3 months of age. Thirty-three feet had a so-called rocker-bottom deformity. All of these feet had been treated with intensive prolonged manipulations and casts; none had had prior surgery. In the series, there were 100 patients with bilateral deformity; in 9 (4.5 percent of these clubfeet), one foot responded to nonoperative treatment, while the other required surgical correction. A significant number of feet represented recurrent deformities after apparent successful correction with nonoperative treatment. The recurrent deformity after prior treatment developed at varying ages, between 6 months and 6 years; in all cases, the first suspicion of a recurrent deformity was "heel-cord tightening."

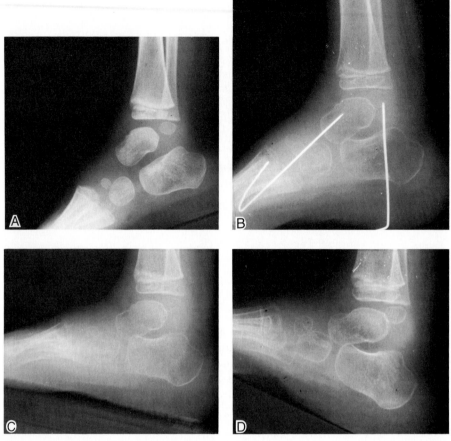

Fig. 7-12. This case illustrates how transfixion of the talocalcaneal transfixion prevents valgus deformity of calcaneus as dorsiflexion is increased in postoperative treatment. *(A)* Preoperative dorsiflexion lateral view at patient, age 3 years and 9 months. *(B)* Six weeks postoperative, dorsiflexion is still limited because the overgrown deformity of the anterior trochlea of the talus impinged on the anterior lip of the tibia. In this case the vertical pin was inserted into the cartilagenous epiphysis of the talus rather than the ossified nucleus. *(C)* The K-wires were removed 10 weeks postoperatively. Dorsiflexion is increased because more of the talus enters the ankle mortise. Note the relationship of the calcaneus and talus is unchanged. *(D)* Five months after surgery full dorsiflexion is possible after remolding of the talus. With transfixion of the talocalcaneal and the talonavicular joints, the talus, calcaneus and navicular move as a single unit as dorsiflexion is increased, avoiding valgus angulation of the calcaneus which may occur when only the talus and navicular are transfixed.

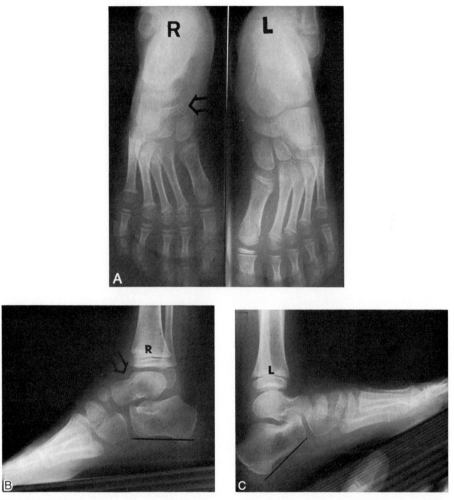

Fig. 7-13.   Illustrative case: soft-tissue release in a 7-year-old. This child had an increasing equinus, cavovarus deformity, after years of treatment with manipulations, plaster and finally a short leg brace. The family had been advised to continue with brace while awaiting a triple arthrodesis at skeletal maturity. At age 7, a Steindler plantar release and a one-stage release were done in one operative procedure. The preoperative radiographs showed typical uncorrected clubfoot deformity (Fig. 7-13*A,B,C*). *(A)* Age 7 years. Anteroposterior view of right clubfoot with comparison view. *(B,C)* Dorsiflexion lateral view. Dorsiflexion is limited. Note anterior trochlea is flat and overgrown.

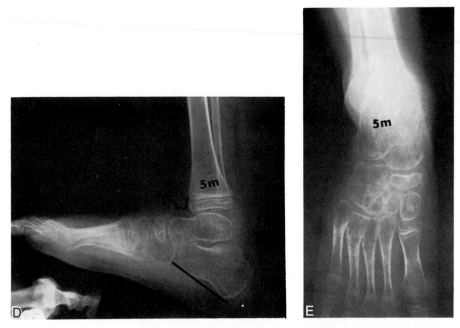

Fig. 7-13. *(continued).*   Postoperatively, dorsiflexion was gradually increased with successive manipulations and cast changes. The internal fixation was removed 2 months after surgery, and plaster immobilization was continued for a total of 5 months *(D,E). (D,E)* Five months after surgery. Lateral view *(D)* shows the remolding of the talus with good dorsiflexion. Anteroposterior view *(E)* demonstrates that the medially displaced navicular is reduced in front of the talar head, divergence of the hindfoot with correction of heel varus.

Age at Surgery.   Age at the time of surgery ranged from 6 months to 8 years; the majority were under 3 years of age. In children 6 to 8 years old, the alternative to soft-tissue surgery was usually a triple arthrodesis at skeletal maturity.

Prior Surgery.   All of the older children had had at least one previous surgical procedure and presented with severe cosmetic and functional deformities. In the series of 273 operations, 104 feet (38 percent) had had one or more previous operations before the one-stage PMR. All the feet with prior surgery had had lengthening of the tendo Achilles, either as the only procedure or concomitantly with other operations, such as posterior release, two-stage medial and posterior release, or lengthening of the posterior tibial and flexor tendons. In the series, 44 patients with bilateral deformity had had prior surgery to both feet. In this group of patients the surgery was successful in only one foot of three patients, one following TAL; two were corrected by soft tissue release operations. The history in the group that had prior surgery was comparable to those that had only nonoperative treatment; some appeared to be corrected temporarily after surgery only to develop increasing deformity that subsequently necessitated another operation.

Failure of previous one-stage PMR operations.   Fifteen feet in this series were failures of prior one-stage PMR done at other centers. Analysis of this group of cases revealed some significant factors regarding the surgical age, the technique,

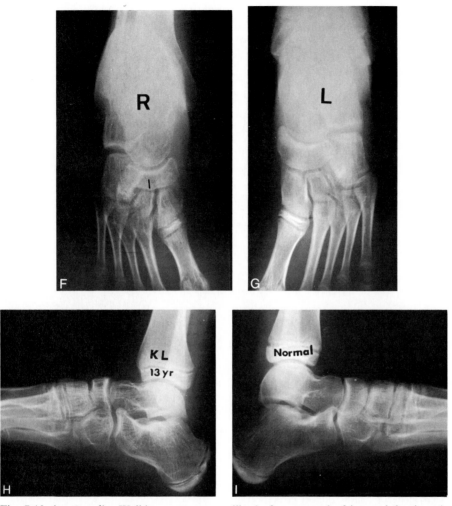

Fig. 7-13 *(continued)*. Walking casts were utilized after removal of internal fixation. A corrective plaster splint was used at night for one year. At 14 years there was slight calf atrophy, supple subtalar motion, dorsiflexion equal to the normal side an excellent athlete. Arthrodesis has been avoided. Radiographs show normal tarsal relationship with slight residual abnormality of the head and neck of the talus *(F,G,H,I)*. *(F,G)* Age 13 years. Radiographs show normal tarsal relationship of navicular and calcaneus with the talus. *(H,I)* Lateral view at 13 years shows dorsiflexion is normal. Note slight abnormal configuration of the head and neck of talus as compared to the normal left foot.

and the importance of the postoperative treatment. Six of these children had surgery at 5 months of age, seven between 6 and 12 months, and two at 24 months. Review of the prior surgical technique and postoperative management revealed that no internal fixation was used in five cases, three were held in plaster for only 2 months postoperatively; and in five, below-the-knee casts were used after removal of the internal fixation. The postoperative care was unknown in two cases.

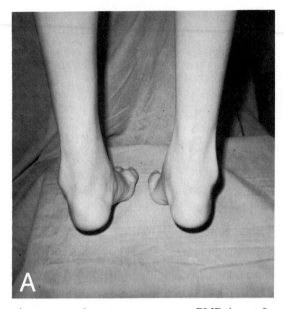

Fig. 7-14. Illustrative case to demonstrate one-stage PMR in an 8-year-old child with bilateral severe equinocavo-varus deformities. Manipulation and cast treatment had been started in the nursery. Previous operations included bilateral TAL at 4 months. Following this operation, the feet "looked good for 4 years." Then the deformity recurred and he wore drop-foot braces. At 6 years of age, bilateral posterior releases were done. Once again, braces were utilized until the equinus deformity precluded continued use of braces. At age 7 years, it was recommended to "wait, return" at maturity for a triple arthrodesis. The deformity and disability increased. The child was first seen at 8 years with severe bilateral foot deformities and hyperextension of the knees. Standing, his heels could not touch the floor. He walked on his toes, with the heels 4 cm off the floor *(A)* and with abduction and genuvalgum of the left leg. At 8 years of age, bilateral one-stage PMR and Steindler plantar release were done. In spite of the severity of the deformity, it was possible to do the Steindler at the same time as the PMR because there were no previous surgical scars along the medial aspect of the foot.

These results suggest that correction must be maintained uninterruptedly for 4 months after surgery. An analysis of the prior treatment demonstrates the advantage of internal fixation and the difficulty of maintaining correction with a below-the-knee cast after removal of the K-wire, especially in a small child under one year of age (Fig. 7-15).

Evaluation of Results

It is difficult to evaluate clubfoot surgery because many preoperative variables can influence the results. These include the severity of the deformity, age of the patient, prior nonoperative treatment, prior surgery, number and type of operations, and iatrogenic abnormalities. In the authors opinion, no completely normal feet result from surgery for resistant deformities; all show some variation from the

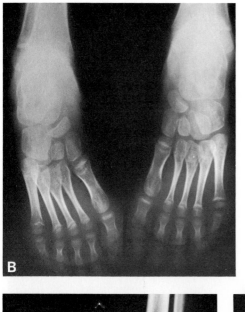

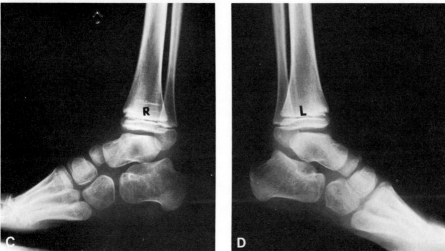

Fig. 7-14 *(continued)*. The preoperative radiographs showed no hindfoot divergence. Medial displacement of the ossified navicular is obvious. *(B)* Lateral views in maximum dorsiflexion revealed severe equinus with "flat-top" tali *(C,D)*.

normal. Clinical examination will show varying residua, such as calf atrophy, asymmetry of foot size, minimal limitation of subtalar mobility, pes planus, metatarsus adductus, or toe-in gait. Even when the results are excellent, critical roentgenographic examination of the talus usually shows some variation from the normal.

Each foot was evaluated cosmetically, functionally, and radiographically, and rated according to the following criteria: *excellent,* i.e., complete correction of all components of the deformity, plantigrade, cosmetically acceptable, pliable subtalar motion, dorsiflexion equal to the normal side or above the right angle in bilateral deformities, and good gait and push-off. Radiographs showed normal tarsal relationship. Results were considered *good* when all components of the deformity were

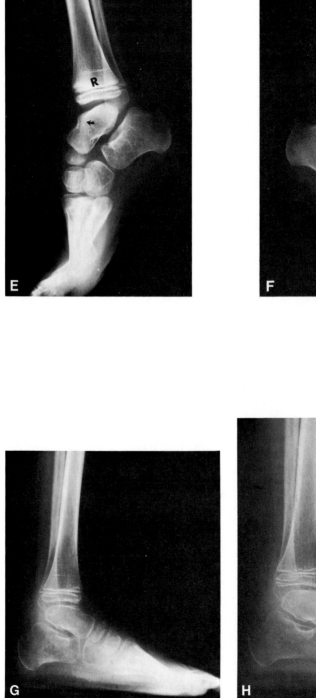

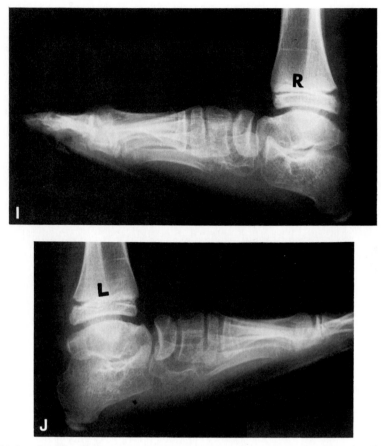

Fig.7-14 *(continued).* Before surgery was undertaken, internal rotation lateral radiographs were made in order to evaluate whether the posterior portion of the trochlea was rounded— a prerequisite for successful soft-tissue surgery in this age group *(E,F)*. Each view, made with the ankle rotated medially shows that the posterior trochlea is rounded. Note how the overgrown anterior trochlea (arrows) and absence of talar neck constriction can block dorsiflexion by limiting the entrance of the body of the talus into the mortise. This view also demonstrates more realistically the severity of the equinus. Initially following surgery, dorsiflexion was quite limited because of the deformed talus. Nine weeks after surgery, the internal fixation was removed. Dorsiflexion had improved following remolding of the tali *(G,H)*. However, residual deformity of the trochleae is still visible. Note change in talocalcaneal relationship in *G* and *H* in comparison to preoperative lateral views. Dorsiflexion was gradually increased at each successive cast change. Plaster immobilization was continued for 5 months following surgery, and walking casts were used after removal of internal fixation. This child incurred an extra articular undisplaced fracture of the right calcaneus while in his last walking cast; a similiar fracture was incurred in the left foot one month after plaster was discontinued. It is believed that both fractures were related to disuse osteoporosis in an active child. Since the subtalar joint was not involved, the fracture healed without any deleterious effect. Two years after surgery, he had one episode of painful peroneal spastic flatfoot that required plaster immobilization for relief of pain. The lateral radiographs at age 14 *(I,J)* show 20° dorsiflexion, round smooth trochleae.

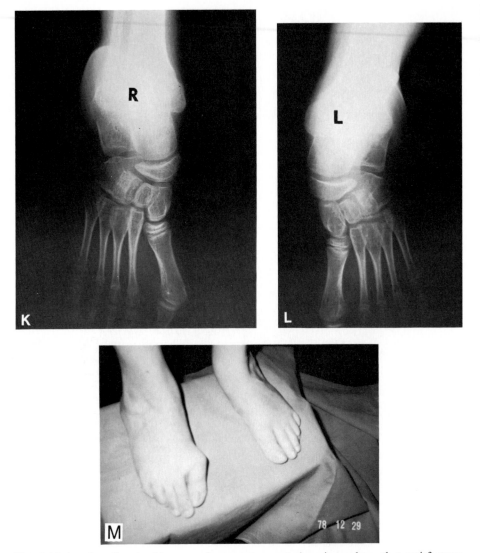

Fig. 7-14 *(continued).* At 14 years of age, anteroposterior views show that satisfactory tarsal relationship has been maintained (Fig. 7-14 *K,L, preceding page*). Soft-tissue surgery was done to minimize deformity of the talus should a triple arthrodesis become necessary, or even hopefully avoid a triple. At this age, the feet are plantigrade, painfree, very serviceable, and cosmetically acceptable. The patient is able to wear regular shoes, including athletic footwear. There is some limitation of subtalar and ankle motion, but this does not impede his gait and activities. Fig. 7.14*(M)* Photograph of the same patient, age 14 years. The right foot developed a hallux valgus with a mild metatarsus adductus primus. Time will determine if the bunion will require surgery. The result is quite satisfactory and far superior to bilateral triples. Triple arthrodesis was avoided, function improved because soft tissue surgery corrected the deformity to allow physiological stimulus for the remodeling of the tali (Fig. 7-14*M*).

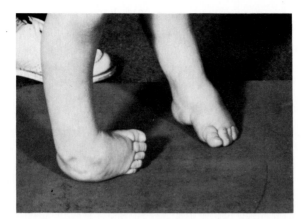

Fig. 7-15. This case is an example of recurrent deformity after one-stage PMR due to inadequate postoperative treatment. Surgery was done at another center at 5 months of age. Postoperatively plaster immobilization was discontinued 2 months after surgery. Surgical correction must be maintained in corrective casts until tarsal bones remold stable articulations.

completely corrected. Radiographic assessment was the same as that for feet in the excellent category but there were one or more mild, cosmetically acceptable residua, such as calf atrophy, asymmetric foot size, pes planus or pliable metatarsus adductus, and toe-in gait. *Fair,* indicated that the feet were plantigrade, functionally acceptable, less acceptable cosmetically, and overcorrection or some loss of the initial correction. The overcorrections had a more severe pes planus, heel valgus, metatarsus adductus, increased dorsiflexion, and limited plantar flexion and subtalar motion. Radiographs showed increased valgus of the hindfoot, lateral placement of the navicular on the talar head, and a closed sinus tarsi. In this category a lasting correction was obtained, function was good, but the feet were less acceptable cosmetically. *Failure* indicates the correction was lost and the deformity recurred. Cosmetically unacceptable planovalgus deformity, due to overcorrection, was also classified as a failure.

Results

The end result is a study on 180 feet with a postoperative follow-up of 2 to 16 years. Utilizing the criteria for evaluation as outlined previously the results were excellent and good in 86 percent; fair in 9 percent; and a failure in 5 percent. Correlating the results with the length of follow-up showed that the correction was maintained, some feet improved with age. Some cases that were initially rated as fair progressed to good and some that were good, became excellent as the children matured. Feet completely corrected 2 years after surgery, stayed corrected. Better results, noted in more recent cases, may be attributed to modifications of the original technique and improved postoperative care. Most of the fair results were overcorrected flatfeet; very few were due to partial loss of correction. All failures except two were due to loss of correction; two were cosmetically unacceptable overcorrections with severe planovalgus deformities. Evidence of recurrent deformity was usually noted within the first year after surgery, and in most cases the loss of correction was either evident or suspected when postoperative plastercast immobilization was discontinued.

Factors Affecting Results

Age at Operation. The best results were obtained in children who were operated on between the ages of 1 and 2 years. Beyond 2 years of age, the number of excellent results diminished as surgical age increased. The incidence of failures was greater in children who had undergone surgery when less than 1 year old. Analyses of 15 feet in the series of failures after a one-stage PMR done elsewhere revealed that in 13 the operation had been done when the child was less than a year old. The higher incidence of failures under age 1 is probably related to the difficulty of maintaining the correction in a small foot after internal fixation is removed. Some surgeons are recommending surgery in infancy;[23,35] the author prefers to operate after the child is a year old for the following reasons: there is a higher incidence of failures when surgery is done under 1 year of age; the small foot is more difficult to maintain corrected in plaster after internal fixation is removed; a minimal error of overcorrection in infancy represents a greater overcorrection than when the same degree of overcorrection occurs in an older child; delayed surgery minimizes the possibility of operating on an unrecognized neuromuscular deformity; surgery is done when the child is walking to take advantage of the normal physiologic stimulus for tarsal remolding; technically, the operation is a little less difficult; and most importantly the long-term results show that earlier surgery has no advantage. Earlier surgery would be advantageous if, at maturity, the radiographs showed evidence of a more normal-shaped talus in children who were operated on when they were less than a year old. To date this advantage has not been evident.

Prior Treatment. The results in feet that had been operated on previously were not as good as in surgically virgin feet, results were best in patients who had only a prior TAL. Considerable scar tissue was encountered in all patients who had had prior surgery; the most extensive scarring usually being noted after tendon-lengthening operations, especially when a K-wire had been used to transfix the calcaneus in plaster. The results were better when the midtarsal joint was found to have been untouched by the previous surgery.

Correlation of the abnormalities noted at surgery with previous nonoperative treatment suggests that some of the abnormal shape of the talus may be acquired iatrogenically by compression or repeated, forceful, prolonged manipulation. Also, there was more fibrosis of the soft tissues in patients who had received more prolonged nonoperative treatment, with manipulations and plaster-cast immobilization.

Usually it is possible to predict a less favorable result when more than the usual primary deformity of the head and neck of the talus is noted at the time of surgery.

Postoperative Care. Loss of surgical correction during postoperative care is often a cause of failure. A review of the postoperative management in this series, and in a group of patients who had had a previous one-stage PMR elsewhere, revealed that many of the failures were due to the failure to maintain surgical correction after internal fixation was removed. Other reasons for unsuccessful results were discontinuation of postoperative immobilization 2 months after surgery; failure of a below-knee cast to hold the correction after internal fixation is removed; and cast slippage. The results of these studies suggest that correction must be maintained without interruption for at least 4 months after surgery.

Overcorrection and Pes Planus. Overcorrection and pes planus usually occur when the navicular is fixed in an overreduced lateral position relative to the head of the talus. This slight error is magnified when the minimal overcorrection occurs in the young infant. Complete transection of the talocalcaneal interosseous ligament will produce a severe pes planus and valgus angulation of the heel and should be avoided; only the amount necessary to unlock the calcaneus and correct the deformity should be transected. Most feet had varying degrees of pes planus immediately after operation. In addition, a bony bulge appears under the medial malleolus; usually these gradually diminish with growth and maturity (Fig. 7-16). The residual pes planus in the excellent and good results was not an aesthetic or functional problem at maturity. The following are prone to flatfeet: a preoperative rocker-bottom clubfoot; more plantar flexion of the talus than usual; and the foot of a child with hyperflexible joints and a flatfoot on the contralateral normal side, when the sustentaculum tali is markedly underdeveloped. Pes planus on the contralateral side of the unilateral deformity is not uncommon and has been seen in feet that were corrected without surgery. A mild degree of pes planus after correction is desirable.

Calf Atrophy and Weakness. The amount of calf atrophy and weakness is related to the extent of lengthening of the tendo Achilles. All patients had considerable weakness and calf atrophy immediately postoperatively, which gradually disappeared as muscle power increased and function returned to normal. The atrophy and weakness was more severe in patients who had had one or more lengthenings of the tendo Achilles, especially when the calcaneus was incorporated in the cast with a K-wire. Calf atrophy and weakness is minimized by avoiding excessive lengthening, as was previously described in the operative technique.

Sectioning or Lengthening of Posterior Tibial and Flexor Tendons

Opinions differ regarding the advantages of lengthening the posterior tibial and flexor tendons. In a series of bilateral deformities under 3 years of age, the posterior tibial tendon was lengthened in one foot and severed in the other. Long-term results to date have shown no appreciable difference between the two sides (Fig. 7-16). Clinical examination of some of the patients years after surgery suggests that the posterior tibial tendon had regenerated; this regeneration was also observed by McCauley.[24] Regeneration of the posterior tibial, Achilles, and flexor tendons has been noted by surgeons during one-stage PMR operations in patients who had had tenotomies at prior operations. In infants, unlike adults, tendons have a

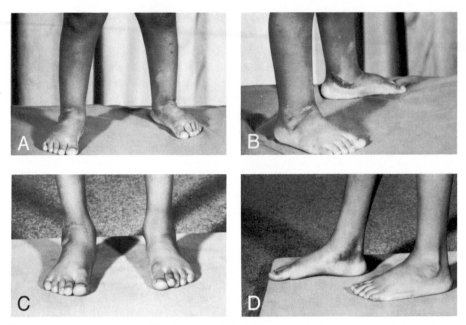

Fig. 7-16.   Illustrative case. This bilateral deformity demonstrates that the initial pes planus and bulge under the medial malleolus usually subside with maturity. This case also compares the results of sectioning and lengthening the posterior tibial tendon. At age one bilateral PMR was done. One the right side the posterior tibial tendon was lengthened, sectioned on the left. Two years postoperatively, he had bilateral pliable pes planus with a bulge under the medial malleolus, which was treated with scaphoid pads *(A,B)*. At 10 years of age *(C,D)*, there was no appreciable pes planus, and the bulge below the medial malleolus had disappeared. The feet were symmetrical in appearance and function *(C)*. No functional or cosmetic deficit resulted from transecting the posterior tibial tendon, and he had a good longitudinal arch bilaterally *(D)*.

greater capacity to reanastomose after sectioning. Therefore, in older children the posterior tibial tendon is lengthened when possible. If the posterior tibial tendon is lengthened, it is recommended that only the insertion on the navicular be left intact; the broad attachments to the spring ligament and sustentaculum tali should be cut to mobilize the navicular and calcaneus.

The flexor digitorum and flexor hallucis longus tendons were not lengthened in this series. Although these muscles are shortened, this does not contribute to the basic pathology; there have been no flexion contractures of the toes. In the long-term, end-result study, temporary flexion of the toes, especially the great toe, is not unusual immediately after surgical correction, because the medial concave border of the foot is lengthened. When the sustentaculum tali is hypodeveloped, the flexor hallucis longus tends to slip into the subtalar joint. In these feet, the flexor hallucis longus was transplanted below the medial malleolus with no appreciable difference in the long-term results.

Calf Atrophy and Weakness.   The amount of atrophy and weakness of the calf is related to the extent of lengthening of the tendo achilles. All patients have considerable weakness and atrophy immediately postoperatively, which gradually improves with time as muscle power increases with the return of normal function. Rarely, if ever, is the size of the calf symmetric in unilateral deformities. Atrophy and weakness are more severe in patients who have had one or more lengthenings of the tendo achilles, especially when the calcaneus had been previously incorporated in the cast with a K-wire. Calf weakness and atrophy have been minimized by avoiding excessive lengthening, as described in the technique.

Wound Complications

In the series of 273 operations, wound dehiscence or skin necrosis occurred in six feet, four of which had been operated on previously. One of these cases had had two previous operations and another had had three previous soft-tissue operations. There were five superficial wound infections. In patients who developed wound complications, satisfactory results were obtained if the foot was maintained in plaster in the corrected position for at least 4 months, which allowed the wound to heal by secondary intention. Plastic surgery is usually not necessary and, if possible, should be avoided. After plastic surgery, invariably the correction is lost, either because the foot is placed in the equinus position to minimize the skin defect or the postoperative dressing fails to maintain the foot in the dorsiflexed position. Ten of the 11 feet complicated by wound problems healed with satisfactory results when the foot was maintained in plaster in the corrected position for 4 months; the scar tissue did not cause a recurrent deformity. One patient with a dehiscence had a recurrent deformity when the foot was placed in the equinus position following plastic surgery.

Metatarsus Adductus—Peroneal Weakness

Varying degrees of pliable metatarsus adductus with toe-in gait are common for a few years after surgical correction. However, these deformities gradually improve and have not been a problem at maturity. Parents must be reassured that toe-in gait usually improves gradually, and at maturity there may be a slight, residual, cosmetically acceptable "pigeon-toe gait," which will not interfere with function. The results in this series concur with the study by Wynne-Davis[46] who noted that metatarsus adductus is not a significant problem at skeletal maturity. To date it has not been necessary to release the tarsometatarsal joints, as described by Heyman and Herndon[20] (Fig. 7-17). I concur with Bleck[4] that increased medial angulation of the neck of the talus plays a role in the toe-in gait. The improvement that gradually occurs with growth after surgical correction can be partially attributed to remolding of the talus; as a result of normal physiologic stress, the increased medial angulation of the neck and talar head is gradually diminished. Increased strength of the peroneal muscles after correction is another factor responsible for diminution of toe-in gait. It is very difficult to evaluate muscle power in infants. In older children, when muscle evaluation is possible preoperatively, many children are found to have weak peroneal muscle strength. In these cases, when the only

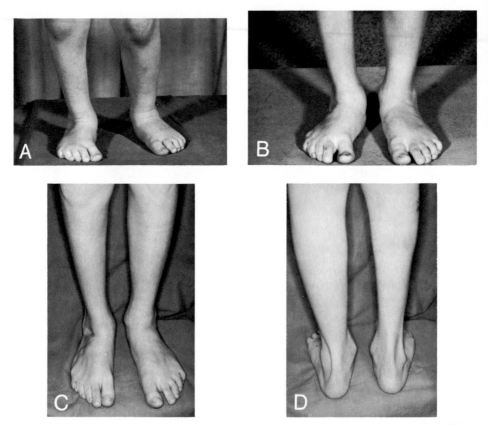

Fig. 7-17. Illustrative case to show that pliable metatarsus adductus subsides. This child had a right clubfoot that had prior posterior release at one year. At 18 months, he had a one-stage PMR. Two years after surgery, *(A)* he had a moderately severe metatarsus adductus with weak peroneals. At 5 years of age *(B),* the adductus was rather severe and cosmetically unacceptable without shoes, marked toe-in gait with weak peroneals. At this time a tarso-metatarsal release was considered but postponed because the forefoot deformity was pliable. With maturity the forefoot deformity gradually subsided with increasing power of the peroneals. At 13 years there was no forefoot deformity and a normal gait *(C,D).*

residual postoperative deformity is a significant pliable metatarsus adductus and toe-in gait, I have observed repeatedly that they gradually subside and that the foot's appearance and gait improve as power returns in the peroneal muscles. This reversible weakness suggests that peroneal palsy is the result, not the cause of clubfeet.

The most severe metatarsus adductus is seen with marked overcorrection of the navicular and valgus angulation of the heels, resulting in the so-called skew-foot (Fig. 7-18). When this deformity is severe and shows no evidence of improving, the foot is treated with a series of manipulations and walking casts to invert the heel and abduct the forefoot. After a short course of manipulations, the child should use a scaphoid pad and Thomas heel for walking shoes; the corrected position is maintained at night with a bivalved corrective cast. Surgery is considered

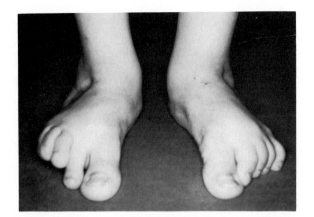

Fig. 7-18. "Skewfoot." Bilateral one-stage PMR done at another center at age 5 months. This illustrates the result of overcorrecting the navicular, and excessive valgus angulation of the heel. This complication is more apt to occur when surgery is done very early.

for a very severe, persistent, and unacceptable skew-foot that fails to improve with nonoperative treatment. In a limited number of these cases the deformity has been minimized by combined lateral and medial soft-tissue release, with percutaneous K-wire transfixion of both the talonavicular and talocalcaneal joints. A Grice procedure with internal fixation is recommended in the older age group for the severest deformities. The rationale of surgery in these severe deformities is to minimize the deformity, or at least prevent further changes in the shape of the tarsal bones should triple arthrodesis be necessary at maturity.

My studies have revealed that overcorrected, unacceptable skewfoot deformities are more apt to occur after soft tissue surgery in the following: cases where the plantar flexion deformity of the talus is exaggerated more than the usual; deformities associated with muscular dystrophy or neurological conditions such as spina bifida; and feet that develop clinical and roentgenographic features of a plantarflexed talus after nonoperative treatment for deformities that appeared as typical indiopathic clubfeet at birth. A severe skewfoot is more disabling and unacceptable cosmetically than a recurrent clubfoot deformity; therefore surgery should be postponed until absolutely necessary in cases that are prone to develop this iatrogenic complication. It is very difficult or virtually impossible to detect the predisposition to skewfoot in infancy; this is one of the reasons I prefer to do a one-stage PMR after 1 year of age, thereby avoiding this potential unsuspected complication.

Peroneal Spastic Flatfoot—Pain

In this series there were 12 patients who had recurrent episodes of peroneal spastic flatfoot. This occurred more commonly with overcorrection in the older age group of surgically treated boys. The more symptomatic feet required a few weeks of manipulation and cast application; all recovered from this malady and became asymptomatic.

Except for pain associated with peroneal spasm and trauma, clubfeet, in children, are usually painless. However, children who develop early wear changes over the anterior tibio-talar joint at skeletal maturity, secondary to the overgrown anterior trochlea and neck of the talus, may experience pain usually localized over the anterior aspect of the ankle. This pain is not common nor is it a cause of prolonged disability; symptoms usually are relieved by temporarily elevating the heel. Postoperatively, fracture of the calcaneus can occur in the older active child while in walking casts. Fractures of the lower tibia and metatarsals have also occurred after removal of the plaster cast. These fractures are due to disuse atrophy.

Hallux Valgus

Hallux valgus is uncommon in clubfoot. When it occurs, it usually does so after skeletal maturity. I have found from my experience, that hallux valgus is more likely to occur in children with the severest deformity, who have had multiple operations. Hallux valgus is often associated with a flexion contracture of the interphalangeal (IP) joint of the big toe, and interphalangeal fusion may be necessary to eliminate the painful callosity and deformity of the IP joint. Hallux valgus has also been observed in the normal foot of a unilateral deformity.

Unusual Findings and Anomalies

In the series of 273 soft-tissue operations, the following unusual findings and anomalies were noted:

1. *Flexor Accessorius Longus.* The flexor accessorius longus is a vestigial anomalous muscle of the foot, described by Grogono and Jowsy[18] in 1965. This accessory extrinsic muscle, located below the posterior neurovascular bundle, was found in 18 of the 273 operations (6 percent). The muscle was attached either on the calcaneus or the intrinsic toe flexor. As the plantaris may or may not be present, the flexor accessorius longus must not be confused with it. The anomalous muscle may be a thin rudimentary structure or quite well developed. We have routinely cut its tendon, and when the muscle was well developed, it was transferred to the achilles. Interestingly, of 8 patients who had bilateral deformities, the anomaly was present bilaterally in only 3.

2. *Absent Tibialis Posterior.* An absent posterior tibial tendon was demonstrated in both feet of 3 patients with bilateral and in the involved foot of 2 patients with unilateral, typical, idiopathic congenital clubfoot. In the patients with bilateral deformity, the tendon was absent bilaterally. Except for the absent posterior tibial tendon, clinical, x-ray, and examination at surgery revealed no other unusual findings. Four additional cases reported to me,[7,21,32,45] were bilateral clubfeet with bilateral absent posterior tibial tendons. The absence of this tendon in idiopathic clubfeet is quite unusual and especially interesting since contracture of this structure is one of the most important, consistent contracture in the resistant clubfoot. The author's experience, added to the cases reported by others, indicates

that a contracted tibialis posterior *per se* is not the prime cause of clubfoot. The results of one-stage PMR in these cases were excellent or good in 7 and a failure in 1. Without the tibialis posterior, the operation is slightly more difficult because the absence of its tendon makes it difficult to exert traction on the navicular. In these cases and those that had previous sectioning of the tibialis posterior, the deltoid attachment is used to distract the navicular from the head of the talus during surgical exposure for the medial release.

    3. *Talocalcaneo Coalition.* This abnormality is not considered likely in club-feet; it is usually associated with a valgus deformity of the heel. In the series of 273 operations, a bar connecting the talus and calcaneus was encountered in the surgery of 13 feet among 8 patients between the ages of 13 months and 8 years. Bilateral ossified coalition has been seen in radiographs of bilateral clubfeet of two additional patients aged 8 and 12 years (Fig. 7-19). Three additional cases have been reported to me. The clinical and x-ray examination of the feet in the surgical series showed no unusual findings to make one suspicious of a different type of deformity; appearance at birth and preoperative assessment were typical of idiopathic deformities. Since the bar connecting the calcaneus and the talus was not ossified in the patients comprising the surgical experience, retrospective assessment of the radiographs failed to show any abnormalities to make one suspect the presence of this coalition. Many had delayed ossification of the cuneiforms. In every case, the bar was found in the region of the sustentaculum tali and

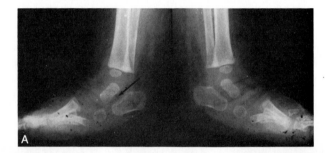

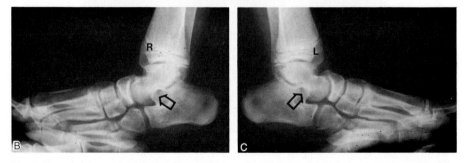

Fig. 7-19. *(A)* Lateral radiographs age 16 months show typical bilateral uncorrected club-feet. The anteroposterior view shows superimposition of talus and calcaneus. Posterior release had previously been done at 18 months for what appeared to be resistant clubfeet. *(B,C)* Oblique views of same patient at 12 years showed osseous talo-calcaneal coalition in the region of the sustentaculum tali.

became evident after the medial contractures were released. Mobilization of the navicular was usually slightly more difficult than usual. The most striking difference in these cases was the difficulty encountered with mobilizing the calcaneus. The calcaneus remained inverted, and its relationship with the talus was unchanged after the posterior release and mobilization of the navicular. It was impossible to evert the heel or distract the calcaneus from the talus, until the coalition was cut.

Talocalcaneal coalition is not to be confused with a fibrocartilagenous mass or scar frequently interposed between the sustantaculum navicular and the malleolus. In the bilateral deformities a coalition was found in both feet of all except one patient. The treatment prior to the one-stage release operation was analyzed in an attempt to ascertain whether the coalition could conceivably be the result of prior treatment. One of the feet had had no treatment whatsoever; 9 had had only nonoperative treatment, and 3 had prior medial release operations. In those patients who had had prior medial soft-tissue surgery, the bar conceivably could be considered the result of iatrogenic changes; however, there was no evidence of articular injury. In 9 of the 11 feet, the coalition was a cartilagenous synchondrosis, which was transected at the time of surgery; in 2 feet, the bar was osseocartilaginous. In all cases, transection was performed easily with a scalpel. The tarsal tunnel and the talocalcaneal interosseous ligament were underdeveloped. To date, the results in these cases has been satisfactory; none have attained skeletal maturity at this time (Fig. 7-20). In the feet that required transection of the coalition, the K-wires were left in place several weeks longer than usual to insure that the subtalar joint remained distracted; weight bearing was also delayed.

4.   *Other Variations.* Minor variations were noted in the relationship and subdivision of the structures that comprise the posterior neurovascular bundle. The findings at surgery demonstrated that in a "simple percutaneous tenotomy" of the achillis tendon it is easy to transect structures other than the achilles because of the deformity and distorted relationship of the contracted structures, in the posteromedial aspect of the foot and ankle.

TENDON TRANSFER

The tibialis posterior and tibialis anterior are the two muscles available for transfer and have been used in selected cases. However, when considering tendon transfer, it is essential to bear in mind the following cardinal principles: a transferred tendon will not correct a fixed deformity; the muscle must be of a sufficient power; and the transferred muscle should pull in a straight line.

Tibialis Posterior Transfer

Fried,[14] Gartland,[16] and Singer[34] have reported on the tibialis posterior transfer in clubfeet for children between the ages of 2½ and 8 years. In this age group, the author prefers to do a soft-tissue release, reserving tendon transfer for selected cases in children over 8 years of age.

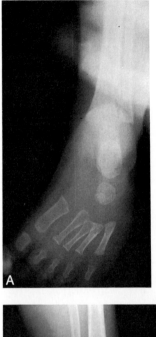

Fig. 7-20.   *(A,B)* Age 2 years. Preoperative radiographs show typical uncorrected clubfoot. Talocalcaneal synchondrosis in the region of the sustentaculum tali was excised, at the time of the one-stage release. *(C)* Age 8 years. Subtalar joint is pliable.

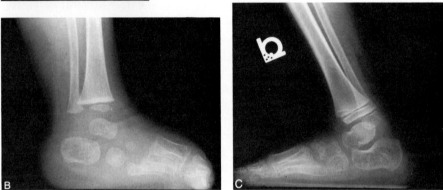

The muscle is transplanted anteriorly through the interosseous space, thereby fulfilling a basic prerequisite for tendon transfer—i.e., pulling in a straight line. The rationale for this operation is to eliminate the deforming force of the contracted tibialis posterior and to utilize its power as a corrective force. The operation should not be done if the goal is to correct a fixed equinovarus deformity. The posterior tibial transfer provides a dynamic, rather than a static, corrective force, and has produced gratifying results in severe toe-in gait. Many of these children readily agree to the operation to avoid the ridicule of their peers, who describe their gait as "walking like a crab." When these feet are examined while the patient is standing, they look quite acceptable, but the unacceptable gait deformity is quite evident when the patient walks.

Indications.   The operation is indicated in children over 8 years of age, who have severe toe-in gait, cavus, weak peroneals and forefoot equinus.

Prerequisites.   While the deformity is not completely corrected, the foot should be plantigrade without severe equinovarus deformity of the calcaneus; the dome of the talus should be well preserved and, preferably, have not had previous medial release. From this description, it is obvious that these feet are incompletely corrected, with mild deformity, and that the chief problem is a cosmetically unacceptable toe-in gait, cavus, and forefoot equinus. If the foot cannot be dorsiflexed to about a right angle, the operation cannot be done because a contracted posterior tibial tendon will not reach the dorsum of the middle cuneiform.

Technique. The posterior tibialis is transferred anteriorly through the interosseous space; a Steindler stripping is usually necessary to correct the associated cavus; and a partial medial release is done as the tibialis posterior tendon insertion is detached.

First incision. A Steindler stripping is done as described previously, through a longitudinal medial plantar incision.

Second incision. To expose the tibialis posterior tendon and the talonavicular joint a second incision is made medially. The posterior tibial tendon then is detached from its insertions on the navicular, the sustentaculum tali, and the spring ligament. At this time, a partial medial release is done and as much correction as possible is obtained, primarily via capsulotomy of the talonavicular joint. The bulbous end of the tendon is narrowed so that the tendon can be passed through the tunnel under the malleolus.

Third Incision. Another incision is made over the medial aspect of the lower leg, through which the posterior tibial tendon is located between the flexor digitorum longus, medially and the hallucis longus, laterally and its distal end delivered. When this transfer is done for peroneal palsy, this incision is unnecessary; the posterior tibial tendon then is delivered through one distal lateral incision. However, the space between the tibia and fibula is quite narrow in the clubfoot and this extra incision facilitates the operation.

Fourth Incision. This incision is made along the lower lateral aspect of the leg. The anterior tibialis is retracted laterally to expose the interosseous membrane, after a window is made through the membrane and it is split proximally by blunt dissection. The tibialis posterior muscle is then transplanted anteriorly through the interosseous space into the fourth wound.

The Last Incision. A final incision is made over the dorsum of the foot in the region of the middle cuneiform, and the tendon transferred subcutaneously under the crural fascia to the dorsum of the foot. A drill hole is made in the middle cuneiform to receive the tendon. However, before the tendon is transferred into the cuneiform, the talonavicular joint is examined and, if necessary to maintain correction, it is transfixed with a K-wire. The posterior tibial tendon is anchored with a Bunnell pullout wire, which is tied over a large button protected from the plantar skin by a piece of felt.

Postoperative Care. The foot is maintained in maximum dorsiflexion in a below-knee cast for 6 weeks postoperatively. After this period of immobilization, the child uses a drop-foot brace for walking and a corrective bivalved cast at night. Children over 8 years of age can usually be taught peroneal exercises; we have not found it necessary to institute physical therapy with muscle reeducation.

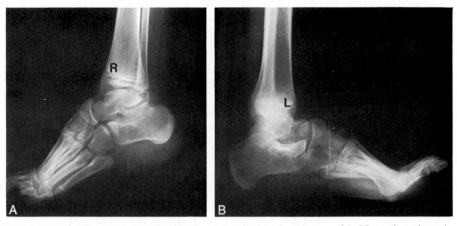

Fig. 7-21. *(A)* Preoperative dorsiflexion lateral view in 12-year-old. Note that there is very little equinus of the calcaneus; most of the equinovarus deformity is in the forefoot. *(B)* Same patient 2 years after surgery, standing view.

The results have been gratifying; patients and their families are pleased because the cosmetically disfiguring gait has been eliminated. Some improvement can be attributed to correction of the cavus component, which contributes to a composite equinus, and the partial medial release, which lessens the varus adduction deformity (Fig. 7-21). In the long-term results, the transfers continue to function well; some children have been able to participate in sports on a competitive level in both high school and college. Some authors have reported that transfer of the posterior tibial results in a cavus deformity due to unopposed action of the anterior tibial and a collapse of the medial border of the foot. I have not noticed these problems following posterior tibial transfer.

Tibialis Anterior Transfer

Transfer of the tibialis anterior laterally, as described by Garceau,[15] is based on the premise that the muscle imbalance caused by a strong anterior tibial with weak peroneals is a deforming factor in clubfoot. Fripp and Shaw[14a] prefer this transfer to the transfer of the tibialis posterior anteriorly. Singer[34] reported: "tibialis anterior transfer had an extremely limited place in the treatment of difficult or relapsed clubfeet." He reported the following undesirable sequel: cock-up deformity of the big toe caused when the disturbed muscle imbalance produced excessive pronation of the forefoot, especially when the tendon was placed too far laterally. My objection to this transfer is that it weakens the major dorsiflexor of the foot, which is already a problem in clubfoot. I prefer to excise the abnormal insertion of the tibialis anterior on the first metatarsal shaft, leaving the normal insertion intact proximally. I would prefer to remove the deforming force of the post-tibialis posterior muscle and to utilize its power as a corrective force.

BONY OPERATIONS

Calcaneocuboid Arthrodesis

The rationale for this operation, as described by Evans,[12] is that the "essential deformity is in the midtarsal joint, other elements of deformity including heel varus are secondarily adaptive." The operation consists of a medial release, a lengthening of the tibialis posterior and tendo achilles, and a wedge resection of the calcaneocuboid joint to shorten the convex lateral border of the foot and stabilize the correction. It is of interest to note that initially Evans[12] recommended that a Thomas wrench be used to correct the cavus component. Lichtblau[23] modified the procedure: he combined a medial release with a lateral wedge excision of one cm. of the distal end of the calcaneus, rather than arthrodesing the calcaneocuboid joint.

Enucleation Procedures

Ogston[28] in 1902 and Codvilla[9] in 1906 mentioned enucleation operations of the cuboid, the anterior part of the calcaneus, and the head of the talus. Results were disappointing, and this method of correction was discarded until Lichtblau modified the technique of the operation described by Evans.[12] Codvilla reported that at the turn of the century enucleation procedures were commonly done; the high incidence of failures prompted him to develop the soft-tissue operation in lieu of bony surgery.

Metatarsal Osteotomies

This surgical procedure has been recommended in older children as a piecemeal operation to correct severe, rigid metatarsus adductus. I have found a limited use for this operation, except in extremely rigid deformities such as arthrogryposis. Metatarsal osteotomies are useful to relieve painful callosities, permit use of a brace or night splint, and also to correct severe forefoot deformity providing the heel is not in excessive valgus.

Osteotomy of the Calcaneus

Dwyer[11] originally described a lateral closing wedge from the calcaneus to correct pes cavus. For the clubfoot, he reversed the procedure and recommended the insertion of a bone graft on the medial side of the calcaneus. Various authors[13,33,44] have reported on the advantages of the medial and lateral approach to the calcaneus, and the advantages of the use of staples for internal fixation. The medial approach stretches the contracted skin in an area notorious for being poorly nourished. Therefore, one should be cognizant of the high incidence of wound problems associated with this operation. This osteotomy is often combined with staged posterior release, posterior tibial transfer, or metatarsal osteotomy.

The proponents maintain that this operation alters the plane of the subtalar joint, as a result weight-bearing exerts a corrective force, and the Achilles tendon is converted to a correcting force. The results I have seen have been disappointing because the operation does not attack the basic deformity in the subtalar and midtarsal joints but only serves to evert the plantar surface of the heel. Calcaneal osteotomy is useful in selected cases, when soft-tissue surgery is impossible or contraindicated. Yet, correction of the varus deformity is mandatory while waiting until a triple arthrodesis can be done.

Osteotomy of the Tibia

A few years ago, the commonly accepted concept was that internal tibial torsion was one of the reasons for "relapse" and toe-in gait. Because of this thinking, external derotation osteotomy was commonly recommended for recurrent deformities that failed to respond to achilles lengthening, posterior release, and two-stage medial and posterior release operations. Presently, external rotation osteotomy of the tibia is rarely adovacated because of the failure to attain satisfactory results. External derotation of the tibia is contrary to our present knowledge of the pathologic anatomy of clubfoot. In general, most investigators agree that excessive lateral rotation of the ankle mortise is present, and this is the reason the fibular appears displaced posteriorly. Singer[34] and recently Lloyd-Roberts[22] and coworkers have again brought to our attention that our former concepts were inaccurate. Based on the concepts of increased external rotation, Lloyd-Roberts has recommended internal rotation osteotomy of the tibia followed by medial soft-tissue release. His preliminary results have been encouraging. The indications for this operation are few and it should be carried out only on selected cases, for the most inveterate deformities where no other procedure is applicable.

Talectomy

With our present-day knowledge and treatment modalities, excision of the talus for idiopathic clubfoot should be rarely necessary. This operation has a place in the treatment of the most severe deformities that have undergone multiple operations when iatrogenic changes in the talus contraindicate soft-tissue surgery and the deformity is so severe that use of orthoses or wearing a shoe are impossible, while awaiting arthrodesis at maturity. The operation should be done under six years of age to allow adaptation of the tarsus with the tibia. After talectomy it is imperative that the foot be maintained plantigrade with an orthosis until maturity. At maturity cosmetically these talectomized feet are quite acceptable, the disadvantages are the loss of leg length and limited ankle motion. This operation has its best indications in the arthrogrypotics, when no other operation will attain a plantigrade foot to allow shoe wearing. This operation also has a place in teratogenic deformities; however, the indication should be questioned in cases in which loss of sensation is associated with spinal cord defects.

TRIPLE ARTHRODESIS

Triple arthrodesis is a salvage procedure that is done at skeletal maturity. The results of routine triple arthrodesis for clubfoot are not good functionally or cosmetically; the deformity of the talus compromises function of the ankle joint. It is our conviction that in this area more should be done with soft-tissue procedures at an earlier age to minimize talar deformity or avoid a triple arthrodesis. Hopefully, the days of advising the 5- to 8-year-old child to "use a brace and return at skeletal maturity for triple arthrodesis" are gone. Standard teaching for residents has been to remove excessive wedges of bone to correct the deformity and attain a plantigrade foot without any concern for cosmetic appearance or the ankle joint. This approach is especially undesirable in the unilateral deformity, where every attempt should be made to attain a cosmetically acceptable foot with the least amount of discrepancy in size.

Many techniques and methods of doing a triple arthrodesis have been described,[29] and, as noted previously, not enough emphasis has been placed on the poor functional and cosmetic results after excessive bone resection. Triple arthrodesis is done when correction by soft-tissue surgery is impossible. There are many borderline cases in which a triple arthrodesis is unnecessary. Examination of adults shows that there are many clubfooted patients whose feet are far from perfect or normal, yet they have little disability or pain. Triple arthrodesis should be considered when the deformity prevents the patient from wearing normal shoes, and to relieve pain caused by callosities and arthritic changes. For the patient who complains of slight pain anteriorly over the tibiotalar joint, relief is possible by using an elevated heel. A triple arthrodesis will not relieve ankle joint pain; on the contrary, ankle pain may be aggravated.

Technique

The goal of triple arthrodesis is to correct the deformity and relieve pain by removing the least amount of bone, thereby minimizing leg length discrepancy and foot size.

Incisions.   Two incisions are made: a medial incision over the talonavicular joint and a linear incision that extends forward just below the tip of the lateral malleolus. Through these two incisions, the talocalcaneonavicular complex is immobilized. An attempt is made to realign the calcaneus and navicular around the head of the talus by mobilizing these bones rather than by excessive wedge resection. Only the articular surface of the head of the talus and the posterior surface of the navicular are denuded to raw bleeding bone. Similiarily, a very thin wafer of bone is removed from the adjacent surfaces of the calcaneocuboid joint and the subtalar joints. It is of interest to note that very little deformity has been found at the calcaneocuboid joint; as expected, most of the deformity is in the subtalar and talonavicular joint. Only a minimal amount of the head and neck of the talus is removed; excessive excision will result in painful impingement of this part of the talus on the anterior lip of the tibia in dorsiflexion. One should not hesitate to fuse the three joints with the ankle in slight equinus, when necessary to prevent impingement in the region of the anterior tibiotalar joint. This slight equinus is readily compensated for by a small heel elevation.

After the navicular is restored in front of the head of the talus and adequate apposition has been obtained in both the calcaneocuboid and subtalar joints, percutaneous K-wires are used to transfix the three joints. These wires are left in place for 6 to 8 weeks, followed by a walking cast until arthrodesis of the three joints is solid. Denuding the articular cartilage and contouring the ball-and-socket configuration of the talonavicular joint produces a better foot cosmetically and also minimizes nonunion, which occurs most frequently at the talonavicular joint.[27]

REFERENCES

1. Attenborough, G. G.: Severe congenital talipes equinovarus. Journal of Bone and Joint Surgery, *46B:*31, 1966.
2. Beatson, T. R.: A method of assessing correction in clubfeet. Journal of Bone and Joint Surgery, *48B,* 1966.
3. Bertelsen, A. Treatment of congenital clubfoot. Journal of Bone and Joint Surgery, *39B:*599, 1957.
4. Bleck, E. E.: Congenital clubfoot-pathomechanics, radiographic analysis and results of surgical treatment. Clinical Orthopedics and Related Research, *125:*119, 1977.
5. Bost, F. C., Schottstaedt, E. R., and Larsen, L. J.: Plantar dissection—an operation to release soft tissue in recurrent or recalcitrant talipes equinovarus. Journal of Bone and Joint Surgery, *42A:*151, 1960.
6. Brockman, E. P.: Modern methods of treatment of clubfoot. British Medical Journal, *2:*572, 1937.
7. Callahan, R. New Haven, Conn. Personal Communication.
8. Carroll, N. C., McMurtry, R., and Leete, S. F.: The pathoanatomy of congenital clubfoot. Orthopedic Clinics of North America, *9:*225, 1978.
9. Codvilla, A.: Sulla Cura Del Piede Equino Varo Congenito: Nuovo Metodo di Cura Cruenta. Arch. Orthop. *23:*245, 1906.
10. Dangelmajor, R. C.: A review of 200 clubfeet. Bulletin of the Hospital for Special Surgery, *4:*000, 1961.
11. Dwyer, F. C.: The treatment of congenital talipes equinovarus by the insertion of a wedge into the calcaneum. Journal of Bone and Joint Surgery, *45B:*67, 1963.
12. Evans, D.: Relapsed clubfoot. Journal of Bone and Joint Surgery, *43B:*722, 1961.
13. Fisher, R. L., and Shaffer, S. R.: An evaluation of calcaneal osteotomy in congenital clubfoot and other disorders. Clinical Orthopedics and Related Research, *70:*141, 1970.
14. Fried, A.: Recurrent congenital clubfoot. Journal of Bone and Joint Surgery, *41A:*243, 1959.
14a. Fripp, A. T. and Shaw, N. E.: Clubfoot. E. & S. Livingstone Ltd., Edinburgh and London, 1967.
15. Garceau, G. J.: Anterior tibial tendon transposition in recurrent congenital clubfoot. Journal of Bone and Joint Surgery, *22:*932, 1940.
16. Gartland, J. J.: Posterior tibial transplant in treatment of recurrent clubfoot. Journal of Bone and Joint Surgery, *45A:*000, 1963.
17. Goldner, J. L.: Congenital talipes equinovarus—fifteen years of surgical treatment. Current Practice in Orthopaedic Surgery, *4:*61, 1969.

18. Grogono, J. S., and Jowsey, J.: Flexor accessoreus longus. An unusual muscle anamoly. Journal of Bone and Joint Surgery, *47B:*118, 1965.

19. Haddidi, H.: Management of congenital talipes equinovarus. Orthopedic Clinics of North America, *5:*53, 1974.

20. Heyman, C. H., Herndon, C. H., and Strong, J. M.: Mobilization of the tarsometatarsal and intermetatarsal joints for the correction of resistant adduction of the forepart of the foot in congenital clubfoot or congenital metatarsus varus. Journal of Bone and Joint Surgery, *40A:*299, 1958.

21. Kleiger, B.: New York, N.Y. Personal Communication.

22. Kuhlman, R. F., and Bell, J. F.: A clinical evaluation of operative procedures for congenital talipes equinovarus. Journal of Bone and Joint Surgery, *39A:*265, 1957.

23. Lichtblau, S.: A medial and lateral release operation for clubfoot. A preliminary report. Journal of Bone and Joint Surgery, *55A,B:*77-84, 1973.

24. Lloyd-Roberts, G. C., Swann, M, and Catterall, A.: Medial rotational osteotomy for severe resistant deformity in clubfoot. Journal of Bone and Joint Surgery, *56B:*37, 1974.

25. Main, B. J., Crider, R. J., Polk, M., Lloyd-Roberts, G. C.; Swain, M., and Kadmar, B. A.: Journal of Bone and Joint Surgery, *59B:*337, 1972.

26. McCauley, J. C.: The history of conservative and surgical methods of clubfoot treatment. Clinical Orthopaedics and Related Research, *84:*25, 1972.

27. McCauley, J. C.: Surgical treatment of clubfeet. Surgical Clinics of North America *3:*561, 1951.

28. Ogston, A.: A principle of curing clubfoot in severe cases in children a few years old. British Medical Journal, *1:*1524, 1902.

29. Patterson, R. L., Parrish, F. F., and Hathaway, E. N.: Stabilizing operations on the foot; a study of the indications, techniques used and end results. Journal of Bone and Joint Surgery, *32A:*1, 1950.

30. Phelps, A. M.: The present status of open incision method for talipes equinovarus. New England Medical Monthly, *10:*217, 1891.

31. Ponsetti, I. V., and Smolley, E. M.: Congenital clubfoot: The results of treatment. Journal of Bone and Joint Surgery, *45A:*261, 1963.

32. Robbins, H.: Personal Communication. New York, N.Y.

33. Salomao, O.: Osteotomia Do Calcaneo Como Tratamento Complementar No Pe Equino-varo Congenito; Faculdade De Medicina Univ. De Sao Paulo, Brasil, 1972.

34. Singer, M.: Tibialis posterior transfer in congenital clubfoot. Journal of Bone and Joint Surgery, *43B:*717 1961.

35. Somppi, E., and Sulamaa, M.: Early operative treatment of congenital clubfoot. Acta Orthopaedia Scandinavia, *42:*513, 1971.

36. Steindler, A.: Stripping of the calcaneus. Journal of Orthopedic Surgery, *2:*48, 1920.

37. Swann, M., Lloyd-Roberts, G. C., and Catterall, A.: The anatomy of the uncorrected clubfoot. Journal of Bone and Joint Surgery, *51B:*263, 1969.

38. Tachdjian, M. O.: Pediatric Orthopaedics, W. B. Saunders, Philadelphia, 1972.

39. Turco, V. J.: Surgical correction of the resistant clubfoot. Journal of Bone and Joint Surgery, *53A:*477, 1971.

40. Turco, V. J.: Resistant congenital clubfoot. Instructional Course Lectures. American Academy of Orthopaedic Surgery, vol. 24, The C. V. Mosby Company, St. Lewis, 1975.

41. Turco, V. J.: Resistant congenital clubfoot—One-stage posteromedial release with internal fixation—a follow-up report of a fifteen year experience. Journal of Bone and Joint Surgery, *61A:*805, 1979.

42. Turco, V. J.: One-Stage Posteromedial Release with Internal Fixation for Resistant

Congenital Clubfoot. Technique Film Library, American Academy of Orthopedic Surgeons, Chicago, Ill.

43. Wagner, L. C., and Butterfield, W. L.: Surgical release of contracted tissues for resistant congenital clubfoot, American Journal of Surgery, *84:*82, 1952.
44. Weseley, M. S., and Barenfeld, P. A.: Mechanism of the Dwyer calcaneal osteotomy. Clinical Orthopaedics and Related Research, *70:*137, 1970.
45. Williams, J. P. Personal Communication San Jose, California.
46. Wynne-Davies, R.: Review of eighty-four cases after completion of treatment. Journal of Bone and Joint Surgery, *46B:*53, 1964.

8 | Nonidiopathic Clubfoot and Other Foot Deformities

FOOT DEFORMITIES

Nonidiopathic talipes equinovarus, talipes calcaneovalgus, plantar-flexed talus, and metatarsus adductus may be part of a systemic musculoskeletal disorder, or the deformed foot may be the only apparent skeletal abnormality at birth. Diametrically opposed deformities in the same patient—such as talipes equinovarus and talipes calcaneovalgus—are usually evidence that the clubfoot is nonidiopathic.

Nonidiopathic Clubfoot. This deformity occurs in genetic syndromes, teratologic anomalies, neurologic disorders of known and unknown etiology, and in myopathies. A child may be born with a congenital predisposition to clubfoot; the deformity develops after birth due to a muscle imbalance, as in neurologic disorders and myopathies. Usually, other stigmata of the skeletal disorder readily distinguish the nonidiopathic deformity. However, in some instances the foot may be the only evident anomaly, in which case the clubfoot, at birth, is often indistinguishable from a typical idiopathic deformity. Clubfoot has been reported in innumerable skeletal syndromes, such as arthrogryposis, nail-patella syndrome, congenital constriction bands, muscular dystrophies, lead poisoning, diastrophic dwarfism, teratogenic anomalies, Gordon syndrome, Mobius syndrome, and many others. Clubfoot is commonly associated with abnormalities of the hands, particularly supernumerary thumbs, eye abnormalities, cleft palate, micrognathia, and delayed motor and mental development. Clubfoot is well known in meningomyelocele, spina bifida, spinal cord defects, and neurologic disorders of unknown etiology.

In some cases, the classic stigmata of any known syndrome are absent, yet the child's facies, the appearance of the foot, and the response to treatment may cause one to suspect a nonidiopathic clubfoot. Usually, a thorough investigation of these cases, including muscle biopsy, enzyme studies, neurologic as well as

167

pediatric evaluation, and genetic studies fails to provide a diagnosis; often the final diagnosis is "a neurologic disorder or a myopathy of unknown etiology."

The discussion of nonidiopathic clubfoot will be limited to a few conditions to illustrate some of the pitfalls in diagnosis and treatment.

Congenital Constriction Bands.   Congenital circumferential constriction bands (Streeter dysplasia) is a rare abnormality that usually involves both the upper and lower extremities. Congenital amputations of the fingers and toes are commonly seen in this condition. In a study of 45 patients with congenital constriction bands, Moses and his colleagues[6] found that 27 percent had a positive family history of congenital anomalies, "chiefly clubfeet." All patients in their series had at least two developmental anomalies, and 14 had clubfoot, which was bilateral in 10.

Clubfoot is commonly associated with congenital amputations of some of the toes, edema, and vascular impairment. Milder deformities respond to manipulation and immobilization in a cast. Soft-tissue surgical correction is recommended for deformities that do not respond to nonoperative treatment. However, before clubfoot surgery, staged "Z" plasty excision of the rings should be done to improve circulation.

In resistant feet, satisfactory results are possible when a one-stage **PMR** is done after plastic surgery on the skin. The postoperative treatment varies in each case, depending on the pathologic findings, especially the degree of skin and muscle involvement. The correction attained by surgery or nonoperative treatment must be protected with corrective night splints much longer than idiopathic deformities (Fig. 8-1).

Hereditary Onycho-osteodysplasia.   This condition, also known as Nail-Patella syndrome, is an hereditary disorder of ectodermal and mesodermal tissues, transmitted as an autosomal dominant gene to both males and females. This syndrome has also been given the eponym of Fong disease,[1] in honor of Dr. E. E. Fong. Fong discovered, in routine pyelographic studies, symmetric bony projections from the posterior aspect of the pelvis, which he called "Iliac horns."

Fong disease is characterized by the absence of patellae and the presence of subluxations of the head of the radii, iliac horns, and nail anomalies. Nail deformities are the most common and most striking abnormalities; changes in the toe- and fingernails may be quite subtle, or show gross obvious abnormalities. The nails may be absent, hypoplastic, or have vertical grooves. Nails on the thumb side of the hand are more involved than those on the ulnar side; the little finger may be normal. Similiarily, the nail of the big toe is most deformed, and the degree of involvement diminishes progressively toward the little toe, which is the least involved or may even be normal. This genetic abnormality can also produce a variety of other deformities of both the upper and lower extremities as well as abnormal pigmentation of the eyes, renal dysplasia, and talipes equinovarus.

The nail deformities may be quite subtle and should cause one to look for other skeletal abnormalities. However, they are characteristic of hereditary onycho-osteo-dysplasia and readily distinguish it from idiopathic clubfoot, arthrogryposis, and other congenital defects. Match[4] reported that 4 of 8 patients afflicted with this syndrome had clubfoot deformities. The milder deformities are amenable to

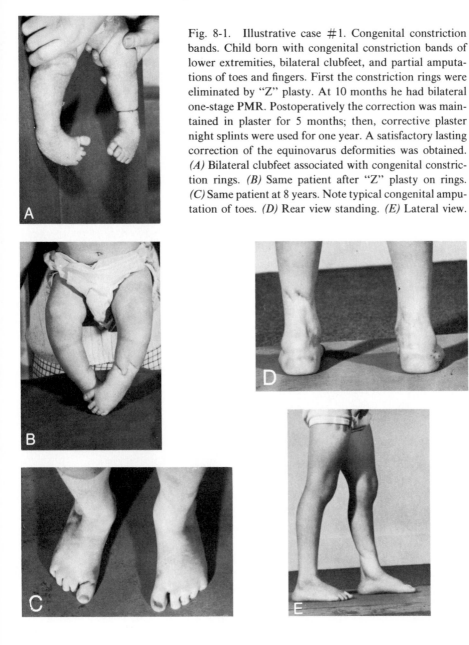

Fig. 8-1. Illustrative case #1. Congenital constriction bands. Child born with congenital constriction bands of lower extremities, bilateral clubfeet, and partial amputations of toes and fingers. First the constriction rings were eliminated by "Z" plasty. At 10 months he had bilateral one-stage PMR. Postoperatively the correction was maintained in plaster for 5 months; then, corrective plaster night splints were used for one year. A satisfactory lasting correction of the equinovarus deformities was obtained. *(A)* Bilateral clubfeet associated with congenital constriction rings. *(B)* Same patient after "Z" plasty on rings. *(C)* Same patient at 8 years. Note typical congenital amputation of toes. *(D)* Rear view standing. *(E)* Lateral view.

manipulation and cast treatment; soft tissue release is recommended for resistant cases (Fig. 8-2).

Arthrogryposis Multiplex Congenita. Arthrogryposis is an uncommon congenital syndrome characterized by muscle wasting, rigid joint contractures, and a high incidence of clubfoot (Fig. 8-3). A common triad includes talipes equinovarus, hyperextension knee contracture, and dislocated hip. In arthrogryposis, the clubfoot

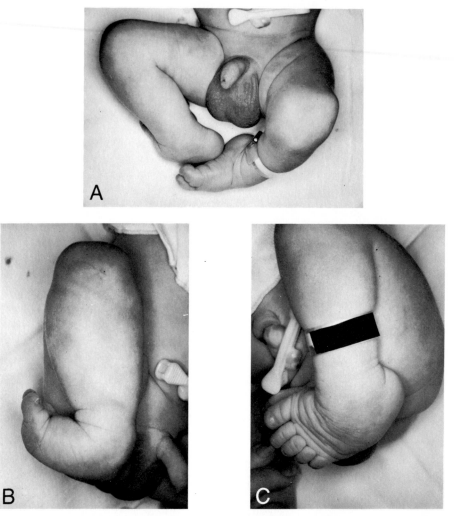

Fig. 8-2.   Illustrative case #2. Nail-Patella Syndrome. Family History—father, brother, and a cousin had the same syndrome; a sister was normal. *(A,B,C)* At birth, this child had typical deformities of toenails and fingernails, absent patellae, bilateral flexion contractures of the knees, a right talipes calcaneovalgus *(B),* and a left equinovarus deformity *(C).* Diametrically opposite foot deformities were pathognomic of a nonidiopathic clubfoot. Manipulation and serial cast treatment was started in the nursery. The right calcaneovalgus deformity was corrected after 12 weeks of treatment. After one year of manipulation and cast treatment, the left foot was plantigrade; however, correction was incomplete. At this time the child used corrective walking shoes and a D-B Bar at night. The result appeared satisfactory for 6 months. Then, the child developed increasing equinovarus deformity. At 2 years he had a one-stage PMR with internal fixation. The posterior tibial tendon was absent.

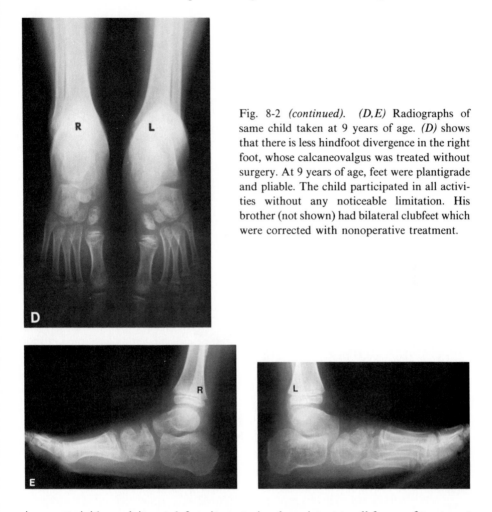

Fig. 8-2 *(continued)*. *(D,E)* Radiographs of same child taken at 9 years of age. *(D)* shows that there is less hindfoot divergence in the right foot, whose calcaneovalgus was treated without surgery. At 9 years of age, feet were plantigrade and pliable. The child participated in all activities without any noticeable limitation. His brother (not shown) had bilateral clubfeet which were corrected with nonoperative treatment.

is a most rigid, recalcitrant deformity notoriously resistant to all forms of treatment and therefore very difficult to correct. Maintaining even partial correction is a challenging problem.

Treatment. Manipulation and plaster immobilization should be started as early as possible. When the hips, knees, and feet are involved, a hip spica is necessary to maintain correction after manipulation of the three areas. The primary goal of treatment is to convert a rigid, deformed foot into a plantigrade foot that will fit into a shoe and is suitable for standing and ambulation. The treatment of choice involves manipulations, serial casting, and corrective orthosis, day and night. Because the results of surgery have been notoriously poor, surgery is performed only when nonoperative management fails to achieve the limited goals of treatment.

Many arthrogrypotic feet are quite serviceable, even though the correction is incomplete. Patients with residual deformity of some of the clubfoot components have a great capacity to adapt to the incomplete correction and are able to function quite well after skeletal maturity. One must constantly keep in mind Sterling Bun-

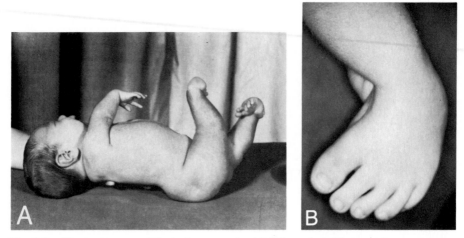

Fig. 8-3.   Illustrative case #3. Arthrogryposis. *(A)* Bilateral clubfeet and hyperextension contractures of the knees. *(B)* Left foot at 6 years after 2 unsuccessful soft tissue operations. Talectomy provided a serviceable plantigrade foot.

nell's adage: "You cannot make a silk purse out of a sow's ear," when treating an arthrogrypotic clubfoot. Multiple surgical procedures are often required to achieve a plantigrade foot, to make it possible for the patient to wear shoes, and to eliminate painful callosities. On occasion, the operative treatment is more radical than the surgical procedure for the idiopathic deformity. When possible, soft-tissue operations are preferable to bony procedures. However bony operations may be necessary and include metatarsal osteotomy, naviculectomy, talectomy, calcaneal osteotomy, and triple arthrodesis. I prefer to avoid a triple arthrodesis, if possible, because many of these patients function quite well with a slight equinovarus, if there are no painful plantar callouses; triple arthrodesis may aggravate the tibiotalar incongruity, which is the result of the abnormal shape of the talus. Often, however, a pantalar arthrodesis may be avoided by doing the triple arthrodesis in slight equinus, thereby permitting limited motion between the tibia and the posterior trochlea of the talus, which is round and better preserved. These patients function quite satisfactorily by wearing a shoe with an elevated heel.

In selected cases, incomplete but satisfactory corrections have been obtained with a one-stage release; the internal fixation should remain in place for several months and postoperative plaster immobilization continued for a longer period of time than for the idiopathic deformity. Due to the high incidence of recurrent deformity especially after soft-tissue surgery, this type of clubfoot must be kept in appropriate orthosis for walking and protected in night splints, until the patient reaches skeletal maturity.

Usually there are other stigmata of arthrogryposis that readily distinguish this clubfoot from the idiopathic deformity. Unfortunately, all clinics have some cases of clubfoot in which all of the characteristics of arthrogryposis are present but the foot deformity is the only area of skeletal involvement; this suggests that this type of apparent idiopathic deformity may represent a *forme fruste* of arthrogryposis. For this reason, the foot does not respond to either operative or nonoperative treatment in the same way that the usual idiopathic deformity responds. In addition to these idiopathic clubfeet, which behave like arthrogrypotics, I have seen cases in which arthrogrypotic-like clubfoot deformities were the only skeletal manifestation of lead poisoning.

It has been noted that clubfeet with short fourth and fifth metatarsal rays are usually more recalcitrant deformities. These deformities have considerable calf atrophy. They look like a localized form of arthrogryposis—a notoriously resistant deformity with a high incidence of recurrence—and respond to treatment similar to arthrogryposis.

NEUROLOGIC DISORDERS

Congenital clubfoot disorders are also associated with many neurologic conditions, such as meningomyelocele, spina bifida, spinal cord defects, hydrocephalus, cerebral palsy, and other ill-defined neurologic disorders[9] (Fig. 8-4).

One should always be suspicious of nonidiopathic deformities when they are asymmetric—e.g., talipes calcaneovalgus on one side and talipes equinovarus on the other side. This is not unusual in myelodysplasia. The author has seen some neurologic disorders that started as talipes calcaneal valgus and later developed

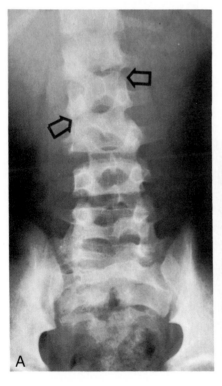

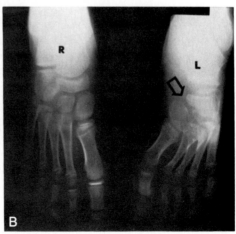

Fig. 8-4.   Illustrative case #4. *(A)* Spinal cord defect. *(B)* Same patient, age 10 years. Left clubfoot deformity recurred after temporary apparent correction following piece-meal operations. Tendency for recurrence is even greater than in idiopathic clubfoot; therefore, the correction must be maintained and protected, especially at night, until skeletal maturity.

into talipes equinovarus. Congenital plantar-flexed talus is often associated with neurologic abnormalities.

Genetic Syndromes. There are many genetic syndromes with skeletal defects that have an associated clubfoot. In fact, clubfeet are common in syndromes with cleft palate, abnormalities of the eyes, micrognathia, and anomalies of the hand, especially of the thumb. Diastrophic dwarfs have clubfeet which are most recalcitrant, resistant, and notorious for their failure to respond to treatment. Often, surgery appears to aggravate deformity.

Teratogenic Deformities. Usually, when a clubfoot is caused by a teratogen, other skeletal defects are visible. It is possible to find cases in which only one foot appears to be involved, as in lead poisoning. However, in these cases all muscles below the knee are severely involved with fibrosis and shortening. Terato-

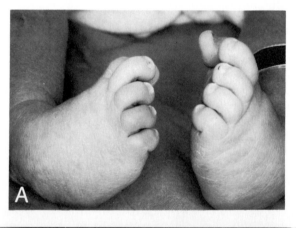

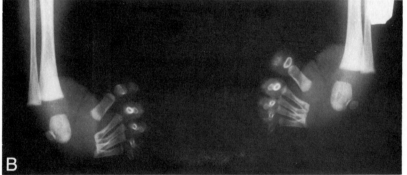

Fig. 8-5.   Illustrative case #5. This case is an example of a child born with what appeared to be idiopathic clubfeet. Subsequently, it became apparent that the talipes equinovarus was in fact due to a neuromuscular abnormality of undetermined origin. This case illustrates the importance of recognizing a nonidiopathic clubfoot in order to avoid iatrogenic complications of surgery which can compound the foot deformity in neuromuscular problems. The child was the product of a full-term, uneventful pregnancy and delivery. At birth, the only apparent abnormality was bilateral clubfeet *(A)*. The clinical and radiographic examination at birth showed findings indistinguishable from typical idiopathic clubfeet *(B)*.

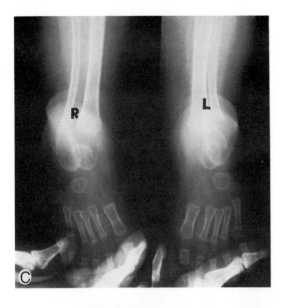

Fig. 8-5 *(continued).* Manipulation and casting were started in the nursery, followed by adhesive bandaging which had to be discontinued because of skin irritation. Initially, the right foot was the more resistant. Evaluation after 3 months of treatment revealed uncorrected resistant feet with a rocker-bottom on the right side (5C,D). Continuation of manipulations was fruitless; therefore, it was decided to use a D-B Bar as soon as the feet were big enough to fit into corrective shoes. It was planned to continue with the DB Bar and passive stretching exercises while awaiting one-stage PMR planned for one year of age.

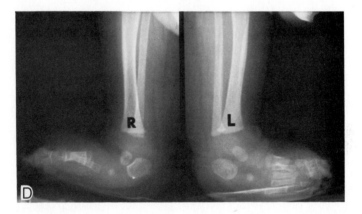

genic problems may also be caused by a viral infection or pelvic inflammatory disease early in pregnancy.

Myopathy. Clubfoot due to muscular dystrophies may be very subtle. At birth, some of these patients appear to be normal except for what appears to be a typical idiopathic clubfoot. However, when the child is between 6 and 12 months of age, it becomes apparent that the problem is due to a musculoskeletal developmental syndrome, often of unknown etiology. Doing a one-stage release early in infancy involves the risk of operating on an unrecognized muscular dystrophy. This is one of the reasons I prefer to delay definitive surgery until the child is a year old. These deformities may begin as typical talipes equinovarus, and during the course of treatment convert to what appears to be a plantar-flexed talus.

In the author's opinion, surgery is preferably avoided or delayed until it is absolutely necessary in the musculodystrophy group. With nonoperative treatment,

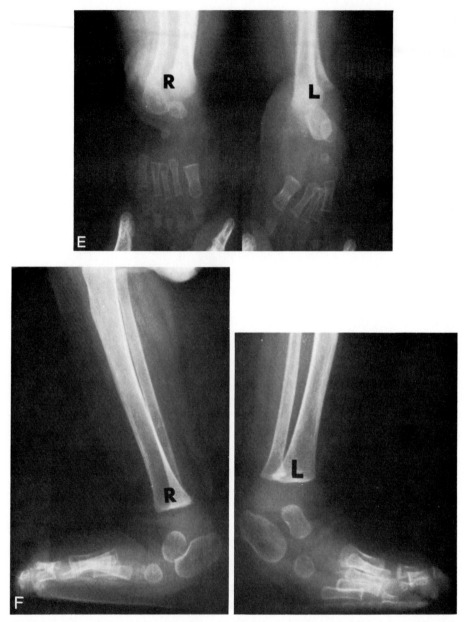

Fig. 8-5 *(continued).*   At 7 months of age, it was first noted that the child's left eye "turned in" and that he had "roving" eye movements. By 8 months of age, it was quite apparent that he had a peculiar facies, delayed motor development, "floppy" muscle tone, a neuromuscular disorder associated with an ophthalmological disorder. Complete work-up with skull and spine radiographs and neurologic and genetic studies shed no light on the diagnosis. Since the clubfeet were not idiopathic, it was decided to defer surgery. At one year of age, the clinical and radiographic examination showed persistent uncorrected clubfeet with some divergence of hindfoot *(E)* and considerable plantarflexion of the tali and calcanei *(F).* Note in *F* that the right foot *(R)* resembles a plantarflexed talus.

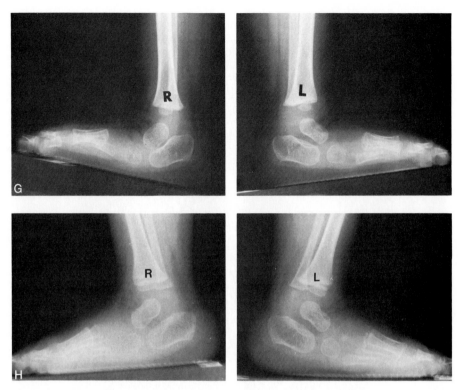

Fig. 8-5 *(continued)*.   At 2 years of age, dorsiflexion improved slightly, but the rocker-bottom persisted on the right side. *(G)*. At age 3, the feet were plantigrade, the rocker-bottom disappeared, and there was less plantarflexion of the tali; however, correction was incomplete, and there was no dorsiflexion of the calcanei (5*H*).

patience, persistence, periodic casting, and the use of orthoses and night splints, these youngsters can function quite satisfactorily in spite of their incomplete correction (Fig. 8-5). Clubfeet caused by muscular dystrophy may appear to correct readily, initially only to recur; or, after prolonged treatment, the heel varus may be overcorrected and the foot may simulate a plantar-flexed talus. These feet are prone to severe, unacceptable overcorrection following a complete posteromedial release. Therefore, surgery should be avoided, or at least postponed, until the deformity becomes static, at which time appropriate surgery can be done, if necessary. In general, talipes associated with myopathies do not respond well to complete soft-tissue release, tendon transfer, or calcaneal osteotomy. All too often following the first surgical intervention, multiple subsequent procedures become necessary to correct iatrogenic problems of surgery. The surgical results are unpredictable and, in general, disappointing. Therefore, before recommending a tibialis posterior transfer to correct a clubfoot deformity, one should ascertain whether the deformity is due to a myopathy and note especially if the talus is markedly plantar flexed. After the tibialis posterior has been transferred anteriorly, these feet often develop

(continued on page 180)

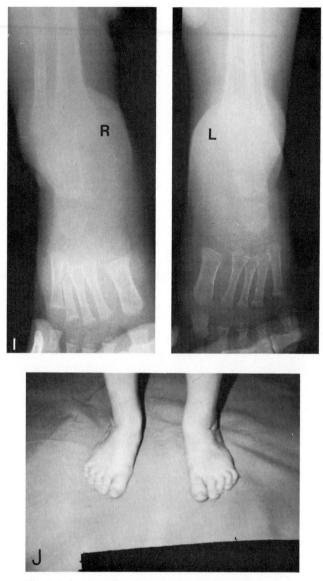

Fig. 8-5 *(continued).* It is significant that at age 3 years the ossification centers of the cuneiforms had not appeared. *(I)* (They usually appear earlier in idiopathic clubfeet.) At age 7, the feet were plantigrade and cosmetically acceptable. Dorsiflexion was limited to 90° and subtalar motion was limited *(J).* At this age, the eye abnormality required bilateral corrective surgery and the wearing of corrective glasses.

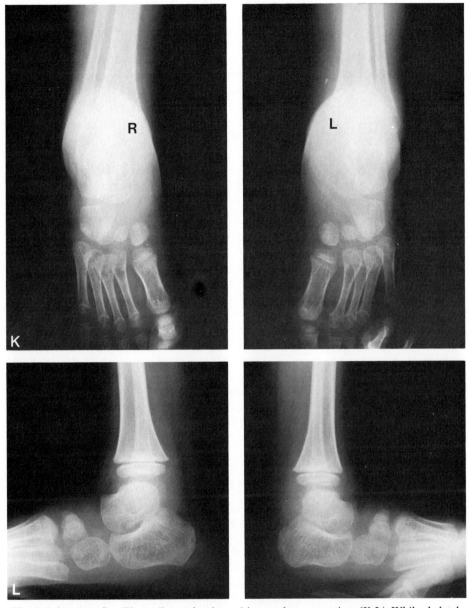

Fig. 8-5 *(continued)*. The radiographs showed incomplete correction *(K,L)*. While skeletal maturity has not been attained, this is a satisfactory result to date considering one is dealing with a neuromuscular disorder. Nonoperative treatment has avoided the bizarre deformities "skewfoot," multiple operations, and possibly eventual triple or even a pantalar arthrodesis necessary to correct iatrogenic deformities which are prone to occur following surgery in neuromuscular clubfeet.

bizarre deformities that usually require multiple corrective procedures and eventually a triple or even a pantalar arthrodesis, with unrewarding results. If soft-tissue release is necessary, care must be taken not to overcorrect the deformity. It is also recommended that the tibialis posterior be lengthened rather than sectioned, to avoid upsetting the tenuous muscle imbalance of these feet. Myopathic deformities do not respond to soft-tissue surgery as well as do idiopathic deformities.

METATARSUS ADDUCTUS—METATARSUS VARUS

These two terms have been used interchangeably to describe a deformity of the forepart of the foot. I prefer to use the term metatarsus adductus when the forefoot is adducted without inversion, and the term metatarsus varus when the five metatarsals are adducted and inverted. The inversion component is usually more prominent in the newborn; by the time most of these children are seen by orthopedists at several months of age, their deformity is usually a metatarsus adductus without a varus component. Occasionally, this deformity has been confused with a clubfoot and has been inaccurately described as "a third of a clubfoot."

Metatarsus adductus is readily distinguished from the clubfoot by: the presence of a normal-shaped heel; the absence of equinus and varus deformity of the heel; a readily visible and palpable posterior tuberosity of the calcaneus on passive dorsiflexion; and well-developed skin creases around the heel (Figs. 8-6*A,B*). The deformity in metatarsus adductus is the result of a forefoot adduction that occurs at the Lisfranc joint without associated adduction at the midtarsal level. Unlike the clubfoot, the midtarsal area and the subtalar joint are usually everted and abducted, and the radiograph shows increased divergence of the hindfoot; in a mild case, the hindfoot may be normal (Figs. 8-6*C,D*).

Incidence

There are no valid statistics concerning the incidence of metatarsus adductus. The general consensus is that the condition is more common than clubfoot but that, unlike clubfoot, it affects both girls and boys equally. However, the incidence appears to be increased in children with a positive family history, many of whom have siblings with the same condition. It is believed that the majority of these deformities clear up spontaneously.[3,6]

Management.   The orthopedist usually sees these children when they are 2 to 3 months of age because of persistent deformity. Their foot deformity should be treated because, in a significant number, it persists. In addition, an unrecognized valgus deformity of the hindfoot, if not properly treated, may result in severe flatfoot. Also, care must be exercised to be certain that treatment does not increase the eversion deformity of the hindfoot. Both parents and siblings should be examined, because many of these children have a hereditary pes planus, some degree of which is to be expected with a positive family history. Hopefully, the pes planus can be minimized with proper treatment. Congenital dislocation of the hip may be associated with ipsilateral metatarsus adductus. For this reason, the hips should

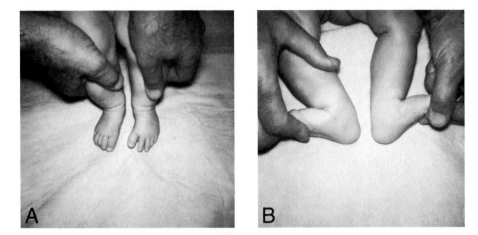

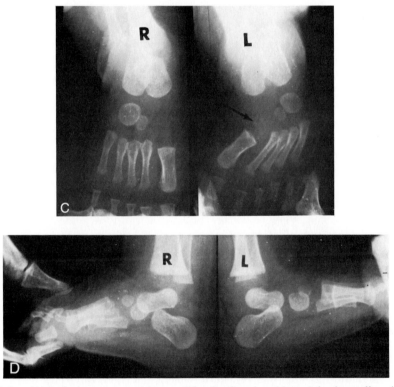

Fig. 8-6. *(A)* Left metatarsus adductus. The forefoot is adducted horizontally without varus. *(B)* Same patient, passive dorsiflexion. There is no equinovarus deformity of the heel. Note the downward excursion of a well defined visible posterior tuberosity of the calcaneus. *(C)* Same patient. Note the adduction deformity of the metatarsals at the Lisfranc area, and increased valgus angulation of the calcaneus of the left foot. *(D)* Dorsiflexion lateral. Unlike the clubfoot, dorsiflexion of the calcaneus is normal in metatarsus adductus.

be carefully examined for tight adductors, limited abduction, positive Ortolani click, and asymmetric deep buttock folds. Radiographs of the hips are taken, if necessary. I have not seen a congenital dislocation of the hip associated with ipsilateral talipes calcaneovalgus except in patients with neuromuscular problems. Nor have I seen a congenital dislocation of the hip together with an idiopathic clubfoot, a common combination in arthrogryposis.

A common combination is the so-called windblown appearance in which one foot has a metatarsus adductus and the other a talipes calcaneovalgus. This is thought to be due to prolonged retention of the fetal position—i.e., the child habitually sleeps in the fetal position, face down. These deformities are usually mild and clear up spontaneously or respond to stretching exercises. However, if this attitude of the feet persists beyond several months or if the parents are concerned, correction is hastened by using an abduction pillow or a turkish towel to keep the hips in the frog-leg position, thereby discouraging the fetal position. Open-toe, tarsopronator shoes may be used in conjunction with an abduction splint and stretching exercises.

Mild Deformities. A mild deformity can be treated with passive stretching exercises and open-toe tarsopronator shoes. In cases with an associated tibia vara, the shoes are attached to a D-B Bar externally rotated 10°. The child's parents should be specifically instructed in the proper method of manipulation. All too often, the mother dorsiflexes the ankle joint and pronates the entire foot; as a result, no effective force is applied at the site of the deformity, namely the tarsometatarsal joints.

Severe Deformities. Manipulation and plaster of Paris immobilization is the treatment of choice for the more severe deformities that fail to respond to the less vigorous treatment outlined above. In manipulation, some pitfalls and iatrogenic problems can be avoided by keeping in mind that these feet have excessive valgus angulation of the heel, and adduction of the forefoot is primarily at the Lisfranc area. Improper manipulation and immobilization can exaggerate the heel valgus and cause a severe flatfoot or, in some cases, subluxing peroneal tendons. This iatrogenic complication has been reported by many authors.[5,7,8]

Exaggeration of heel valgus with a severe flatfoot can be avoided by treatment in which knowledge of the normal mechanics is applied. In plantar flexion, the calcaneus inverts and the navicular moves medially. Therefore, for both manipulation and immobilization, the foot should be held in the equinus position. This position serves to correct the existing valgus angulation and also locks the calcaneus under the talus; thus, the forefoot adduction can be corrected without the danger of increasing heel valgus. During manipulation, the foot is maintained in plantar flexion and the forefoot is forced into abduction while counterpressure is being maintained laterally over the calcaneocuboid joint.

Following repeated manipulations, the foot is immobilized in equinus, maximum forefoot abduction with an above-knee cast. The cast is molded to maintain the forefoot in the corrected position while the plaster is setting. The above-knee cast is necessary to prevent slippage with the foot in equinus. Manipulation and immobilization in equinus avoid the dangers of flatfoot and increased hindfoot valgus, which are more apt to occur when the foot is manipulated and immobilized in the neutral or dorsiflexed position. Since this method has been used, severe flatfoot after treatment has not occurred.

The casts are changed at 2- to 3-week intervals, depending on the patient's age and growth rate. These patients usually require 6 to 8 weeks of immobilization in a plaster cast. After the deformity is corrected, open-toe tarsopronator shoes are worn at night for 4 to 6 months and straight-last walking shoes for 1 to 2 years.

Persistent Severe Deformities.   In general, most cases of metatarsus adductus, exclusive of those associated with arthrogryposis, teratogenic, and skeletal syndromes, respond to the management outlined above. Occasionally, a more severe deformity fails to respond to this treatment. These children usually have a so-called "Z" deformity with more severe planovalgus and forefoot adduction. Clinically, the deformity may appear to be supple and correctable. However, the apparent correctability by manipulation is the result of the adducted forefoot accompanying the abduction of the midtarsal and subtalar joint. This can be documented by radiographic studies. The anteroposterior view, taken with the foot held in abduction, will confirm the valgus exaggeration of the hindfoot and the midtarsal area, while the forefoot adduction persists. Since many improve with growth, a mild or moderate deformity is acceptable and can be treated with appropriate corrective shoes.

Surgery is recommended only for severe, persistent deformities. The recommended operations are capsulotomies of the tarsometatarsal joints[3] and metatarsal osteotomies for the severest rigid deformities. Irrespective of whatever operation is contemplated, it is essential that the degree of heel valgus be considered as an integral part of this problem. In some cases, a Grice procedure may be considered to correct the hindfoot. The forefoot adduction usually responds to manipulation after the hindfoot valgus has been corrected. In a limited experience, satisfactory results have been obtained by correcting the subtalar and midtarsal deformities with soft-tissue surgery. Postoperatively, this correction was maintained with percutaneous K-wire transfixion of the midtarsal and subtalar joints for 10 weeks followed by plaster-cast correction for 5 months. The forefoot adduction was corrected with postoperative manipulations after correction of the valgus angulation of the hindfoot. At surgery, the tibialis posterior had a minimal attachment on the navicular tuberosity with an extensive insertion on the bases of the first and second metatarsals; the talonavicular capsule deltoid and spring ligaments were lax, and the sustentaculum tali was displaced laterally. Surgical intervention should be delayed until after 4 years of age because most of these children will improve. Also, the delay allows time for bony developmental anamolies to manifest themselves.

TALIPES CALCANEOVALGUS

Talipes calcaneovalgus is characterized by dorsiflexion of the foot without any forefoot deformity. The foot appears to be normal except for extreme hyperdorsiflexion. At birth, the dorsal surface is in close proximity to the lower anterior aspect of the leg. The degree of limitation of plantar flexion and the rigidity of

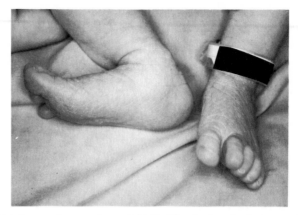

Fig. 8-7.   Right talipes calcaneovalgus at birth. The heel and plantar surface of the foot appear normal. It is significant to note the absence of a convex bony prominence on the plantar surface, which is a distinguishing characteristic of congenital vertical talus.

the dorsal structures, which resist downward movement and inversion of the foot, are variable, the anterior tibial is contracted. The deformity may be unilateral or bilateral; the feet are often quite long (Fig. 8-7).

Incidence.   The incidence of talipes calcaneovalgus is greater in large babies, breech presentations, and babies born to primigravida. This natal history suggests that the deformity is probably caused by intrauterine pressure; however, neuromuscular conditions, especially spina bifida, should be excluded. The radiographs show hyperdorsiflexion of the foot without a breech or forefoot abnormality.

Diagnosis.   It is important to distinguish talipes calcaneovalgus from a congenital vertical talus (congenital convex pes valgus (Fig. 8-8). The latter is often associated with other congenital abnormalities and has a guarded prognosis, as compared to talipes calcaneovalgus, which usually has an excellent prognosis. Plan-

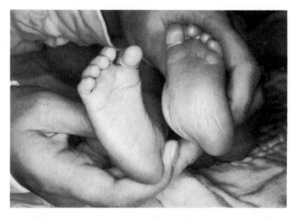

Fig. 8-8.   Left congenital convex pes valgus. Note the convex prominence of the plantar surface, valgus of the heel, forefoot abduction. This patient had a spinal cord defect.

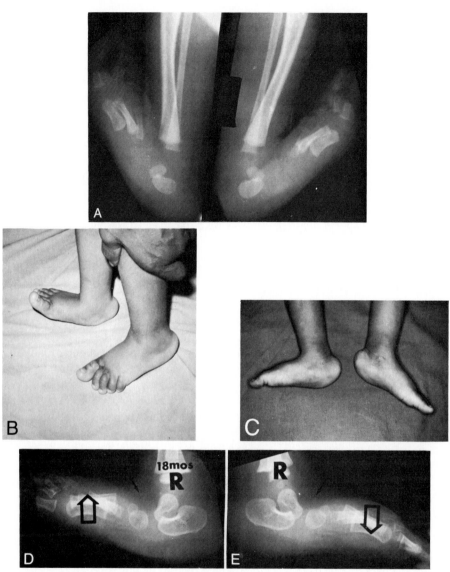

Fig. 8-9. An example of acquired plantarflexed talus. Child was born with bilateral talipes calcaneovalgus documented by radiographs and description on the clinical record. Stretching exercises were recommended. The child was seen at one and a half years of age with bilateral plantarflexed tali more deformed and resistant on the right side, which subsequently required soft tissue release. Manipulation and plaster treatment at birth would have most likely avoided surgery and produced a better result. *(A)* Radiographs at birth show typical calcaneovalgus deformities. Dorsiflexed position of calcanei distinguish this from congenital vertical talus. *(B,C)* At one and a half years, acquired bilateral plantarflexed talus. Deformity is more severe on right side. Note convex bulge on plantar surface, and severe planovalgus with forefoot abduction of the right foot. *(D,E)* Radiographs of right foot at 18 months with right foot held in maximum dorsiflexion *(D)* and plantarflexion *(E)*. Note that the talus remains unchanged in the same vertical position, the dorsal concavity of the foot is also unaffected by forced dorsiflexion and plantarflexion. Also note that unlike the typical congenital vertical talus, plantarflexion of the talus is oblique rather than vertical.

tar-flexed talus is caused by a dorsolateral dislocation of the talocalcaneonavicular complex; the navicular is displaced dorsally and the calcaneus is in equinus and everted. Rigid contractures of the anterior deltoid ligament, dorsal part of the talonavicular capsule, anterior tibial, extensor tendons, and the Achilles resist correction of this deformity. Congenital plantarflexed talus is a very rigid deformity with the following indistinguishable typical features: the forefoot is fixed in dorsiflexion and abduction, causing a dorsal concavity; a convex bony prominence on the plantar surface represents the unsupported exposed head of the talus; and the heel is fixed in equinus and valgus with the posterior tuberosity of the calcaneus quite prominent (Fig. 8-8). A number of methods of correction have been proposed for this notoriously resistant deformity.

Treatment.   Many mild deformities tend to correct themselves spontaneously or with passive stretching. If the deformity at birth is severe, the treatment of choice is manipulation and plaster-cast immobilization. Complete correction and immobilization in full equinus on the first treatment in the nursery is precarious because the skin over the dorsum of the foot is contracted and the danger of skin necrosis is magnified by the bow-stringing effect of the tibialis anterior. For this reason, initially I prefer to manipulate these feet daily and maintain the correction by applying an ace bandage over cast padding. After the foot is loosened and the skin and contracted tendons are partially stretched, a plaster cast is applied, maintaining the foot in the maximum degree of equinus and varus with sufficient cast padding over the dorsum to avoid pressure sores. In the serial manipulations, the equinus and varus are gradually increased until correction is complete. Several months of manipulation and plaster-cast immobilization are usually required. The Denis Browne bar is used for 4 to 6 months after the deformity is corrected by manipulation and plaster casting. When these children begin to walk, they usually have pronated feet that may require corrective shoes.

Most of these deformities correct themselves without treatment. However, I have seen cases that at birth were typical talipes calcaneovalgus progress to a plantar-flexed talus. These are cases that develop a plantarflexed talus after birth secondary to acquired soft-tissue contracture (Fig. 8-9). Giannestras[2] feels that many cases of talipes calcaneovalqus are predisposed to pes planus. While it is true that many of these deformities correct spontaneously, the author regretfully had been lulled into complacency by this past thinking. However, I am no longer mesmerized by this philosophy, as I now feel these deformities, in the newborn, should be watched more carefully. If there is any question of a rigid, persistent deformity beyond a few days, I prefer to treat the deformity more vigorously with manipulation and casts. Early treatment is innocuous, usually successful, and considered a relatively minor inconvenience that prevents the acquired deformities noted above.

REFERENCES

1. Fong, E. E.: Iliac horns-symmetrical bilateral central posterior illiac processes. Radiology, *47:*517, 1946.

2. Giannestras, N. J.: Recognition and treatment of flatfeet in infancy. Clinical Orthopaedics and Related Research, *70*, 10, 1970.
3. Heyman, C. H., Herndon, C. H., and Strong, J. M.: Mobilization of the tarsometatarsal and intermetatarsal joints for the correction of resistant adduction of the forepart of the foot in congenital clubfoot or congenital metatarsus varus. Journal of Bone and Joint Surgery, *40A:*299, 1958.
4. Match, R. M.: Onycho-osteoarthrodysplasia with equinovarus. New York State Medical Journal, *73:*1105, 1973.
5. McCauley, J., Lusskin, R., and Bromley, J.: Recurrence in congenital metatarsus varus. Journal of Bone and Joint Surgery, *46A:*525, 1964.
6. Moses, J. M., Flatt, A. E., and Cooper, R. R.: Annular constricting bands. Journal of Bone and Joint Surgery, *61A:*562, 1979.
7. Ponsetti, I. V., and Becker, J. R.: Congenital metatarsus adductus. Journal of Bone and Joint Surgery, *48A:*702, 1964.
8. Rushforth, G. F.: The natural history of hooked forefoot. Journal of Bone and Joint Surgery, *60B:*530, 1978.
9. Tachdjian, M. S.: Pediatric Orthopaedics. W. B. Saunders, Philadelphia, 1972.

Index

Page numbers followed by "f" represent figures

Abductor hallucis muscle, 19, 55
Achilles repair and postoperative mobilization, 119-120, 115f
Achilles tendon, 115
  lengthening and posterior capsulotomy of, 116, 114f
Adduction, 45
  of forefoot at Lisfranc level, 64f
Adhesive strapping, 95-96, 98f
Age at surgery, 112, 148
Angle distortion in radiologic evaluation, 63-64, 68f-69f, 71f
Ankle
  in clubfoot, 43-44
  normal
    and foot, joints of, 24-27
    ligaments of, 25
Arthrodesis
  calcaneocuboid, 160
  triple, 135, 162-163
Arthrography in clubfoot, 63
Arthrogryposis
  in bony operations, 160-161
  clubfoot as, 7
Arthrogryposis multiplex congenita, 169, 171-173, 172f

"Baby fat," 93, 123, 106f
Bony operations, 160-161
  arthrogryposis in, 172
Braces and splints, nonoperative, 95-96

Calcaneocuboid arthrodesis, 160
Calcaneofibular ligament, 25
Calcaneus bone
  in clubfoot, 49, 50
    displacement of, 48f
  normal, 19-21, 20f
  osteotomy of, 160-161
  and talus, abnormal relationships between, 61f

and tibia, abnormal relationships between, 61f
Calf and extrinsic muscles in clubfoot, 55-56
Calf atrophy and weakness, 149, 150-151
Callous, 125, 129f
  on dorsal aspect of fifth metatarsal, 39, 40f
Cast(s)
  above-knee, 122f
  applying, 90
  caring for, 91-92
  long leg, 90, 91f
  removing, 91
  slippage of, postoperative, 123-124, 122f-124f
  walking, 141f
    below-knee, 124, 125f
Cavus deformity, 55, 55f, 72-73, 77f
  operative technique in patients with severe, 131, 132f
Cavus in clubfoot, 45
Chopart's (midtarsal) joints, 25-26, 51
Chubby feet, 121, 106f-107f
Clubfoot
  ankle in, 43-44
  deformity in
    components of, 44-45
    nature of, 37-39, 40, 37f-39f
    osseous, 45-51, 47f-49f, 51f
  etiology of, 5-15
    arrested fetal development in, 8-10
    genetic counseling and, 11
    heredity in, 10
    heredity plus intrauterine environment in, 10-11
    mechanical factors in utero in, 6
    neuromuscular defect in, 7-8
  flexible versus rigid, 7, 38, 38f
  history of, 1-3, 8-9, 35

Clubfoot *(continued)*
  incidence of, 11-14
    demographic statistics and, 12
    family history and, 13-14
    laterality and, 13
    personal series and, 12
    sex ratio and, 12-13
  knee and lower leg in, 42-43, 43f
  nonidiopathic, 167-168
    versus idiopathic, 6
  normal ossification versus, 59
  pathognomonic signs of idiopathic, 40-44,
    42f, 43f
  pathologic anatomy of, 44-56
    in skeletal syndromes, 167
  skin abnormalities in, 39-40, 41f
  soft tissue contractures in, 51-56, 52f-55f
  treatment of
    nonoperative. *See* Nonoperative treat-
      ment of clubfoot
    operative. *See* Operative treatment of
      clubfoot; PMR—personal series
"Congenital clubfoot," definition, 6
Congenital constriction bands, 168, 169f
Congenital convex pes valgus, 184, 184f
Congenital defects versus teratologic defects,
  5
Congenital dislocation of the hip, 10
"Congenital" versus "genetic," 5
Congenital vertical talus, 184, 184f
Constrictions, congenital (Streeter dyspla-
  sia), 168, 169f
Cuboid bone
  in clubfoot, 49, 51
  normal, 24
Cuneiforms and metatarsals in clubfoot, 51

D-B bar (Denis Browne bar)
  as holding splint, 100, 104, 101f,
    102f-103f
  in metatarsus adductus, 182
  in nonoperative treatment, 93-94, 94f,
    99f
  in postoperative treatment, 124, 125f, 175f
  in TAL, 103, 104f
  in talipes calcaneovalgus, 186
D-B splint (Denis Browne splint), 95, 97f
Deformity(ies)
  increasing, 98, 100, 131
  recalcitrant, 137
  recurrent, 98, 99f
    after one-stage PMR, 147f
Deltoid ligament, 25
Denis Browne bar. *See* D-B bar

Enucleation procedures, 160
Equinocavus deformity, severe, internal fixa-
  tion in, 136f-137f
Equinus, cavovarus deformity, increasing,
  139f
Equinus in clubfoot, 44-45

Fat legs and thighs, 121, 123, 122f
Feet, chubby, 121, 106f-107f
Fetal development in clubfoot etiology, 8-10
Fibrosis in clubfeet, 7
Fixation, internal. *See* Internal fixation
Flexible versus rigid clubfeet, 7, 38, 38f
Flexor accessorius longus, 154
Flexor digitorum longus
  and flexor hallucis longus, in clubfoot, 54
  normal, 18
Flexor hallucis longus
  in clubfoot, 54
  normal, 17-18
Flexor tendons, sectioning or lengthening of,
  149-151, 150f
"Floppy" child, 87
Fong disease, 168-169, 170f-171f
Foot, normal, 17-33
  and ankle, joints of, 24-27
  bones of, 19-24
  in maximum dorsiflexion, 22f
  movements of, 28-33
    adduction-abduction of forefoot, 33
    dorsiflexion and plantar flexion, 30-33,
      31f, 32f
    eversion, 30, 30f
    horizontal, 27, 28, 27f
    inversion, 28-30, 29f
  muscles of, 17-19
  radiograph of, 29f
Foot anatomy, pathologic, 35-57
  varying abnormal findings in, 36-37
  varying concepts of, 35-36
Foot deformities, 167-173
Forefoot adduction at Lisfranc joint, 180

Gastrocnemius muscle, 17
Genetic counseling in polygenic hereditary
  conditions, 11
Genetic syndromes with skeletal defects,
  174
"Genetic" versus "congenital," 5
Genuvalgum, 43-44, 44f
Germ plasm defect, primary, 8, 46

Hallux valgus, 154
Heel, inversion of, 39, 39f

Heel-cord
  shortening of, 94
  tightness of, 124, 137
Hereditary onycho-osteodysplasia, 168-169,
  170f-171f
Heredity in clubfoot etiology, 10
  intrauterine environment plus, 10-11

Increasing deformity, 98, 100, 131
  equinus cavovarus, 139f
Infancy, radiographs during, 60-62, 61f
Internal fixation, 118-119, 115f, 140f, 141f
  advantages of, 133-35, 136f-137f, 138f
  personal series, one-stage PMR with, 137,
    140-143, 147-156
  in severe equinocavus deformity, 136f-
    137f
Intrauterine environment in clubfoot etiol-
    ogy, 8-9
  heredity plus, 10-11

"K" wires (Kirschner wires), 118-119, 120,
  138f
  calf atrophy and weakness and, 151
  in one-stage PMR, 142
  in postoperative care, 120, 123-124, 122f
  in tendon transfer, 158
  in triple arthrodesis, 163
Knee and lower leg in clubfoot, 42-43, 43f

Leg, lower, and knee, in clubfoot, 42-43,
  43f
Lisfranc joint, 26
  forefoot adduction at, 180, 64f
  hypermobility at, 70, 75f

Manipulation in nonoperative treatment, 88-
  90
  frequency of, 91-92
  in metatarsus adductus, 182-183
Master knot of Henry, 18, 115
Meningomyelocele, 87
Metatarsal osteotomies, 160
Metatarsals and cuneiforms in clubfoot, 51
Metatarsus adductus (or metatarsus varus),
  180-183, 181f
  and peroneal weakness,
    151-153, 152f
Midtarsal joint, 25-26, 51
Muscle and tendon attachments, abnormal,
  56
Muscular dystrophies, clubfoot due to,
  175, 177, 180, 174f-179f
Myopathy, 175, 177, 180, 174f-179f

Nail-patella syndrome, 168-169, 170f-171f
Navicular bone
  dorsal subluxation of, 121f
  in clubfoot, 49, 51f
  normal, 24
Naviculocuneiform joint, 26
Neonatal examination in nonoperative treat-
    ment of clubfoot, 87-88
Neonatal period, radiographs in, 59-60,
    88, 60f
Neurologic disorders, 173-180
Neuromuscular defect in clubfoot etiology,
    7-8
Newborn, nonoperative primary treatment
    of, 88
Nonidiopathic clubfoot and other foot
    deformities, 167-186
Nonoperative treatment of clubfoot
  borderline corrections in, 94-95
  evaluation at two to three months of age
    in, 92
  initial visit with parents in, 85-86
  methods of, 86-87
    adhesive strapping, 95-96, 98f
    braces and splints, 95-96
    manipulation, 88-90, 91-92
    plaster of Paris casting, 90-92, 91f
  neonatal examination in, 87-88
  primary treatment of newborn in, 88
  in resistant foot, 100-107
  results of, 96-100
  successful, 92-94
Numerical measurement of talocalcaneal an-
    gles, 63-64

Onycho-osteodysplasia, hereditary, 168-
    169, 170f-171f
Operative treatment of clubfoot, 109-
    163
  advantages of internal fixation in,
    133-135, 136f-137f, 138f
  age at operation in, 112, 148
  bony operations in, 160-161
  intraoperative assessment of correction in,
    132-133
  PMR (one-stage posteromedial release
    with internal fixation) in. *See* PMR;
    PMR—personal series
  postoperative care in, 120-135
    guide to, 120-131, 121f-130f
    for older child, 132-133
  review of techniques in, 109-111
  in severe cavus deformity, 131, 132f

Operative treatment of clubfoot *(continued)*
  soft-tissue release in older children
    in, 135, 139f-141f, 142f-146f
  tendon transfer in, 156-159, 159f
Osseous deformities in clubfoot, 45-51, 47f-49f, 51f
Ossification centers in clubfoot at birth, 59
Ossification in clubfoot and normal foot, 59
Osteotomy
  of calcaneus, 160-161
  metatarsal, 160
  of tibia, 161
Overcorrection and pes planus, 147, 149, 150f

Peroneal spastic flatfoot, 153-154
Peroneus longus and peroneus brevis muscles, 19
Pes planus
  in metatarsus adductus, 180
  overcorrection and, 147, 149, 150f
Pes valgus, congenital convex, 184, 184f
"Pigeon-toe gait," 151
Plantar aponeurosis muscle, 19
Plantar calcaneonavicular ligament (spring ligament)
  in clubfoot, 54
  normal, 26, 27f
Plantar-flexed heels, 103
Plantar-flexed talus, acquired, 186, 185f
Plantar stripping, Steindler, 131, 135, 132f, 139f, 142f
Plaster of Paris casts. *See* Cast(s)
Plaster splint, 95, 96f, 99f
PMR (one-stage posteromedial release with internal fixation), 111-120, 124-125, 131, 126f-127f, 135f, 175f. *See also* Operative treatment of clubfoot; PMR—personal series
Achilles repair and postoperative immobilization in, 119-120, 115f
  advantages of, 133, 134f
  indications for, 112
  internal fixation in, 118-119, 115f
  results of, 111
  technique of, 112-118, 114f-115f
PMR-personal series, 137, 140-143, 147-156
  in absent tibialis posterior, 154-155
  in flexor accessoreus longus, 154
  in hallux valgus, 154
  in metatarsus adductus and peroneal weakness, 151-153, 152f
  in peroneal spastic flatfoot and pain, 153-154

  results in, 147-148
    evaluation of, 142-143, 147
    factors affecting, 148-149
  sectioning or lengthening of posterior tibial and flexor tendons in, 149-151, 150f
  in talocalcaneal coalition, 155-156, 155f
  wound complications in, 151
Polygenic hereditary conditions, genetic counseling in, 11
Polygenic hereditary theory of clubfoot etiology, 12
Posteromedial release. *See* PMR; PMR—personal series
Postoperative treatment, inadequate, 150-151, 147f

Radiographs
  during infancy, 60-62, 61f
  in neonatal period, 59-60, 80, 60f
Radiology in clubfoot, 59-83
  reliability of, 63-70, 64f-69f, 93f
  technique of, 66, 70, 68f-69f
Recurrent deformity, 128f
Resistant foot
  definition of, 100
  nonoperative management of, 100-107
Rigid feet, 103
  flexible versus, 7, 38, 38f
Rocker-bottom deformity, 70, 72, 137, 74f-76f, 121f, 175f
  management of, 102f-103f

Skeletal defects, genetic syndromes with, 174
Skeletal syndromes, clubfoot in, 167
"Skewfoot," 152-153, 153f
Skin abnormalities in clubfoot, 39-40, 41f
Skin clefts, 40, 103, 41f
Skin creases, absent, 42, 87, 42f
Soft-tissue contractures, 51-56, 52f-55f
  medial plantar, 53-55, 53f
  plantar (cavus), 55-56, 55f
  posterior, 52-53, 52f
  subtalar, 54-55, 54f
Soft-tissue release, 139f
  in older children, 135, 139f-141f, 142f-146f
Soleus muscle, 17
Spastic flatfoot, peroneal, 153-154
Spina bifida and clubfoot, 7
Spinal cord defect, 173f
Spring ligament (plantar calcaneonavicular ligament)
  in clubfoot, 54
  normal, 26, 27f

"Spurious correction," 92
Steindler plantar stripping, 131, 135, 132f, 139f, 142f
Streeter dysplasia, 168, 169f
Subtalar joints, 25
Surgical treatment. *See* Operative treatment of clubfoot; PMR; PMR—personal series
Sustentaculum tali bone, 20, 21, 20f

TAL (tendo Achillis lengthening), preliminary, 100, 103-104, 107, 104f-105f, 106f-107f
prior, and one-stage PMR results, 148
Talectomy, 161
Talipes calcaneovalgus, 183-186, 184f-185f
Talipes equinovarus, 1-2, 6
definition of, 37
in rabbit, 7
typical left, 37f
Talocalcaneal angles, numerical measurement of, 63-64
Talocalcaneal coalition, 155-156, 155f
Talocalcaneal joints, 25
Talocalcaneal relationship, normal, 62-63, 62f
Talocalcaneal transfixion, 138f
Talocalcaneonavicular joint, 26-27, 27f
Talocalcaneonavicular socket, lateral subluxation of, 28, 30f
Talofibular ligaments, 25
Talonavicular and subtalar articulations, 23f
Talonavicular capsule in clubfoot, 54
Talus
acquired plantarflexed, 186, 185f
and calcaneus, abnormal relationships between, 61f
in clubfoot, 46-49, 47f, 48f
secondary changes in, 48f
congenital vertical, 184, 184f
flat-top, 73, 76-77, 82, 78f-80f
reversibility in, 77, 81f-82f
normal, 21-23, 22f, 23f
Tarsal bones, 19-24
Tarsal relationship, abnormal, 45f
Tarsometatarsal (Lisfranc) joints, 51
Tarsopronator shoes, 94, 100, 124, 94f, 125f
in metatarsus adductus, 182

Tendo Achillis lengthening (TAL), preliminary, 100, 103-104, 107, 148, 104f-105f, 106f-107f
Tendon and muscle attachments, abnormal, 56
Tendon transfer, 156-159, 159f
Teratogenic agents and fetal environment and development, 9-10
Teratogenic defects or deformities, 174-175
versus congenital defects, 5
Tibia
and calcaneus, abnormal relationships between, 61f
in clubfoot, 43
osteotomy of, 161
Tibial muscle, anterior, 19
Tibial tendon
absent posterior, 154-155
sectioning or lengthening of, 149-151, 150f
Tibialis anterior transfer, 159
Tibialis posterior muscle
in clubfoot, 53-54
normal, 18-19
Tibialis posterior transfer, 156-159, 159f
Tibiotalar joint, 24-25, 22f
"Tight heel cord," 94
Toe-in gait, 151
Triple arthrodesis, 135, 162-163
Trochlea of talus, 21-22
deformity of, 48-49

Unilateral deformity, clubfoot versus normal foot in, 64-66, 64f-67f
Uterine pressure and clubfoot etiology, 6. *See also* Intrauterine environment in clubfoot etiology

Varus in clubfoot, 45

Walking, benefits of, 94

"Z" deformity, planovalgus, 183
"Z" lengthening of tendo Achillis, 116, 114f
"Z" plasty, congenital constriction rings, 168, 169f
"Z" plasty of Achilles, repairing, 120